African Histories and Modernities

This book series serves as a scholarly forum on African contributions to and negotiations of diverse modernities over time and space, with a particular emphasis on historical developments. Specifically, it aims to refute the hegemonic conception of a singular modernity, Western in origin, spreading out to encompass the globe over the last several decades. Indeed, rather than reinforcing conceptual boundaries or parameters, the series instead looks to receive and respond to changing perspectives on an important but inherently nebulous idea, deliberately creating a space in which multiple modernities can interact, overlap, and conflict. While privileging works that emphasize historical change over time, the series will also feature scholarship that blurs the lines between the historical and the contemporary, recognizing the ways in which our changing understandings of modernity in the present have the capacity to affect the way we think about African and global histories.

More information about this series at
http://www.palgrave.com/gp/series/14758

Francis Dube

Public Health at the Border of Zimbabwe and Mozambique, 1890–1940

African Experiences in a Contested Space

palgrave
macmillan

Francis Dube
Department of History, Geography, and Museum Studies
Morgan State University
Baltimore, MD, USA

African Histories and Modernities
ISBN 978-3-030-47534-5 ISBN 978-3-030-47535-2 (eBook)
https://doi.org/10.1007/978-3-030-47535-2

This Palgrave Macmillan imprint is published by the registered company Springer Nature Switzerland AG.
The registered company address is: Gewerbestrasse 11, 6330 Cham, Switzerland

To my family and friends

Preface

Growing up on the Zimbabwean side of this border region, I was always struck by the networks of interdependence that still pervade it. I wanted to dig deeper into the history of the Zimbabwe-Mozambique border to investigate how pivotal it has been in shaping the historical process in the region. Many villagers still have families, across the border, and in many cases, men have wives on both sides of the border. The border, in some places, is just marked by a few strands of falling barbed wire fence. Villagers cross it every day without even realizing it. Many villagers have fields on both sides of the border and cross it for many reasons. Many villagers on Mozambican side of the border region do not even have Mozambican identification. They have more in common with Zimbabweans than other Mozambicans. They use Zimbabwean currency and were severely affected by the economic downturn in Zimbabwe, which resulted in hyperinflation in the 1998–2008 decade. As the Zimbabwean government constantly issued new banknotes (bearer checks) while disowning the older ones in order to keep up with inflation, culminating in the adoption of the multi-currency system in 2008, these Mozambican villagers often found their bags of older Zimbabwean notes worthless. Unlike Zimbabweans, who could quickly exchange the older notes for newer ones, these Mozambican villagers found the wealth they had stored in this Zimbabwean currency disappear. This is just one case of interdependence. There still are many other networks of interdependence, including travel to hospitals, to find healers, and for healers to find medicines and visit patients.

I am grateful to a number of people who helped make this project successful. I want to thank the anonymous reviewers for their invaluable input. At the University of Iowa, special thanks go Professor James L. Giblin and Professor Paul R. Greenough. Many thanks also go to my colleagues at Morgan State University for their support and encouragement.

In Zimbabwe, many thanks to the faculty and students in the Economic History and History Departments at the University of Zimbabwe, particularly. I also extend my gratitude to a number of research assistants in the Economic History Department for helping in collecting oral histories. Many thanks to the staff at the National Archives of Zimbabwe for their invaluable assistance.

In Mozambique, I particularly want to thank Dr. Benigna Zimba of the Department of History at Universidade Eduardo Mondlane in Maputo and the hard-working staff at the Arquivo Histórico de Moçambique and other governmental departments.

I also want to thank my family and friends who have always provided moral and logistical support. My wife, Kate, and my daughters, Kundiso and Rumbidzai, have always been supportive. I, however, take responsibility for any errors and omissions.

Contents

Abbreviations

ABCFM	American Board of Commissioners for Foreign Missions
BSAC	British South Africa Company
FRELIMO	Frente de Libertação de Moçambique
GHI	Government Health Inspector
NC	Native Commissioner
NLV	Native (African) Lay Vaccinator
RENAMO	Resistência Nacional Moçambicana
WHO	World Health Organization

CHAPTER 1

Introduction

The 2014–2015 Ebola epidemic in West Africa highlighted the trans-border nature of epidemics, created in part by the movement of people across borders, and the challenges posed by trans-border coordination of surveillance. Yet this is by no means a new challenge. Portuguese and British colonial governments in Southern Africa, for instance, also dealt with the same public health challenges posed by a common border. The border and the fear of diffusion of diseases it generated contributed to the evolution and implementation of discriminatory public health programs among the Shona people of the Mozambique (Portuguese East Africa)-Zimbabwe (Rhodesia/Southern Rhodesia) border region where mobility was the norm.[1] In this region, mobility was the norm because of environmental diversity and kinship connections, which prompted the need for villagers to access resources that lay across the border and to visit kin.[2] For the colonial governments, cross-border movements of people,

[1] The names Zimbabwe and Southern Rhodesia/Rhodesia are used interchangeably in this book. The same applies to Mozambique and Portuguese East Africa. Other countries discussed in this book are Malawi (Nyasaland) and Zambia (Northern Rhodesia). The portion of Mozambique under study, central Mozambique, was governed by the chartered Mozambique Company for much of the period under analysis, from 1890 to 1942, while Zimbabwe was under British South Africa Company rule from 1890 to 1923, when Responsible Government took over.

[2] The choice of fieldwork sites for this study reflects an attempt to include these different environmental zones, including micro-environments, upland plateaus, lowlands, areas of

F. Dube, *Public Health at the Border of Zimbabwe and Mozambique, 1890–1940*, African Histories and Modernities,
https://doi.org/10.1007/978-3-030-47535-2_1

livestock, and wildlife heightened fears of disease diffusion, which affected health and economic productivity. These administrations therefore implemented invasive public health measures, including border controls, compulsory quarantine, medical inspections or examinations, surveillance measures, vaccinations, as well as colonial suppression of indigenous healing practices. Yet, for African villagers and migrants, the border crossing was a crucial part of their livelihood. Africans therefore contested the colonial governments' public health policies on border restrictions and surveillance. Public health at the border became an area of contestation because of the discriminatory implementation of public health measures and the particularly oppressive nature of settler colonialism, which conspired to make life difficult for Africans. This ultimately contributed to low compliance with invasive aspects of colonial public health and medicine. This contestation of the border and public health by Shona villagers, town dwellers, and migrants served as a powerful force in the constitution of colonial power.[3] Hence, by focusing on the contestation of public health at the border, *Public Health at the Border* explores the utility of the border as a theoretical, methodological, and interpretive construct for understanding colonial public health.

The Zimbabwe-Mozambique border was particularly significant for health, given that cattle disease scares of the turn of the twentieth century, such as East Coast Fever, among others, show how Rhodesians regarded Portuguese East Africa as a reservoir of infection and regarded the

high and low rainfall, and various zones of flora and fauna. The area under focus in Zimbabwe stretches from Pungwe River in the north, down to where the Save River crosses into Mozambique. Its western edge is demarcated by the Odzi and Save Rivers in Zimbabwe and it encloses the Mutare, Chimanimani, and Chipinge districts. In Mozambique, it roughly encompasses the western portions of Manica, Sussundenga, and Mossurize districts. This border region generally falls into areas inhabited by the eastern Shona people, with the Manyika in the north and the Ndau in the south. The major urban centers are Mutare (Umtali), Penhalonga (a gold mine), Chipinge (Melsetter/Chipinga), and Chimanimani (originally a sub-district of Melsetter district) in Zimbabwe. The major towns on the Mozambican side are Manica (Macequece/Masekesa/Massi-Kessi), Espungabera (Spungabera) in Mossurize (Musirizwi Umselezwe/Umsilizi/Mossurise) district, and Sussundenga. While this book focuses on the period from 1890 to 1940, it also includes occasional references to the pre-1890 and post-1940 periods.

[3] Eric Allina-Pisano, 'Borderlands, Boundaries, and the Contours of Colonial Rule: African Labor in Manica District, Mozambique, c. 1904–1908,' *International Journal of African Historical Studies* 36, 1 (2003), pp. 59–82.

Portuguese themselves as incompetent guardians of colonial health.[4] Hence, this anti-Latin prejudice on the part of British in Zimbabwe was a factor that made this particular border appear especially dangerous for public health.

Apart from this colonial rivalry, this historical and cultural context also demonstrates how the conjunction of a particular colonized society, a distinctive kind of colonialism and a particular territorial border, generated reluctance to embrace public health. The border led to the disruption of networks of interdependence, not only economic, but those of kinship in particular. This adversely affected African health, given the fact that decisions about therapy alternatives in many precolonial African societies were made collectively by groups of kin.[5] Some of these Africans in turn challenged colonial public health decisions on who or what could cross the border and when to cross the border and under what circumstances. Thus, certain colonial circumstances impeded the acceptance of therapeutic alternatives that were in fact embraced by colonized people elsewhere.

Public health implies the duty of government to provide for the health of its citizens, a situation which many believe has never been fully realized in Africa.[6] More specifically, public health is the science and art of disease prevention, prolonging life, and fostering physical health and efficiency through organized community efforts.[7] Such efforts are generally preventive in nature and they include sanitation, control of contagious infections, hygiene education, early diagnosis and preventive treatment, and maintenance of adequate living standards. Public health interventions require an

[4] See, for example, Francis Dube, "'In the Border Regions of the Territory of Rhodesia, There is the Greatest Scourge …': The Border and East Coast Fever Control in Central Mozambique and Eastern Zimbabwe, 1901–1942," *Journal of Southern African Studies* 41, 2 (2015): 219–235.

[5] Steven Feierman and John M. Janzen, introduction to *The Social Basis of Health and Healing in Africa* (Berkeley: University of California Press, 1992), 18.

[6] Ruth J. Prince, "Introduction: Situating Health and the Public in Africa," in *Making and Unmaking of Public Health in Africa: Ethnographic and Historical Perspectives*, ed. Ruth J. Prince and Rebecca Marsland (Athens: Ohio University Press, 2014), 1–2. See also Milcah Amolo Achola, "The Public Health Ordinance Policy of the Nairobi Municipal/City Council 1945–62," in *African Historians and African Voices: Essays presented of Professor Bothwell Allan Ogot*, ed. E. S. Atieno Odhiambo (Basel: P. Schlettwein Publishing, 2001), 115, and Maryinez Lyons, "Public Health in Colonial Africa: The Belgian Congo," in *The History of Public Health and the Modern State*, ed. Dorothy Porter (Amsterdam: Rodopi, 1994), 357.

[7] Michael H. Merson et al., *International Public Health: Diseases, Programs, Systems, and Policies* (Gaithersburg: Aspen Publishers, 2001), xvii–xxx.

understanding not only of epidemiology, nutrition, and antiseptic practices but also of social science. However, in colonial Zimbabwe and Mozambique, one essential component of public health, education, was largely absent. Many Shona people of the border region only remember being forced to submit to public health measures without any clear explanation of the purpose of such measures. In view of the fact that they were more coercive than they were persuasive, colonial medical services did little to stimulate changing idioms for comprehending suffering.[8] This also reflects the pitfalls of not implementing organic ideas and the overreliance on health care policies developed in Europe and linked to the process of capital accumulation and political domination.[9] This oppressive nature of colonial medicine extended all the way to the colonial apparatus involved in the manufacture and application of drugs, for example, Lomidine, a drug that the French forced on Africans in their territories, which was later found to be ineffective in preventing trypanosomiasis.[10]

Public health interventions limited people's freedoms of movement, association, and choices of therapies and medical providers and included a host of other dehumanizing effects which were not limited to colonial subjects.[11] Nevertheless, what made the colonial situation unique were questions over the legitimacy of colonial authority and the discriminatory nature of public health programs. In the Zimbabwe-Mozambique border region, these also included colonial repression of indigenous healing practices and values which conveyed and reinforced underlying ideas about health and healing. For Africans, therefore, the blatant refutation of these values constituted "cultural disinheritance."[12] As a result, these indigenous healing practices survived because Africans selectively absorbed and adapted elements of Western biomedicine which appeared useful, just in

[8] Jonathan Sadowsky, *Imperial Bedlam: Institutions of Madness and Colonialism in Southwest Nigeria* (Berkeley: University of California Press, 1999), 116.

[9] Jean-Germain Gros, *Healthcare Policy in Africa: Institutions and Politics from Colonialism to the Present* (Lanham, Rowman & Littlefield, 2016), 40.

[10] Guillaume Lachenal, *The Lomidine Files: The Untold Story of a Medical Disaster in Colonial Africa* (Baltimore: Johns Hopkins University Press, 2017), 5.

[11] For instance, after his treatment in a hospital in Paris, France, in 1929 stricken with pneumonia, George Orwell recounted how doctors and students performed procedures on him without even talking to him. See George Orwell, "How the Poor Die," http://orwell.ru/library/articles/Poor_Die/english/e_pdie (8 August 2014).

[12] George Oduor Ndege, *Health, State, and Society in Kenya* (Rochester: University of Rochester Press, 2001), 1–2.

the same way Europeans internalized some elements of indigenous healing practices.[13]

Questions on the legitimacy of oppressive settler colonial governments, replete with massive land dispossession, forced labor, excessive taxes, and restrictions on movement, among other things, contributed to a lack of trust in colonial institutions and consequently low or noncompliance with public health among the Shona. In the recent past, noncompliance has been used to refer to the measurement of sub-optimal uptake of medical treatment due to a patient's resistance, ignorance, or cultural beliefs, and characteristics of the disease.[14] However, Paul Farmer, looking at the failure of tuberculosis treatments in Haiti, has challenged placing the blame on a patient's beliefs and attitudes. He argues that what are at play are often times "structural barriers" to treatment, such as lack of access to medical care, medical infrastructure, and income.[15] My usage of this term acknowledges the failure of therapy as a result of both material barriers and cultural factors, but goes beyond therapy intake to include all forms of

[13]Tracy J. Luedke and Harry G. West, "Healing Divides: Therapeutic Border Work in Southeast Africa," in *Borders and Healers: Brokering Therapeutic Resources in Southeast Africa*, ed. Tracy J. Luedke and Harry G. West (Bloomington, IN: Indiana University Press, 2006), 4. See also Jean Comaroff and John Comaroff, *Of Revelation and Revolution. Volume Two, The Dialectics of Modernity on a South African Frontier* (Chicago: University of Chicago Press, 1997), 364, Adam Mohr "Missionary Medicine and Akan Therapeutics: Illness, Health and Healing in Southern Ghana's Basel Mission, 1828–1918," *Journal of Religion in Africa* 39 (2009): 437, Francis Dube, "Medicine without Borders: the American Board of Commissioners for Foreign Missions in central Mozambique and eastern Zimbabwe, 1893–1920s," *OFO: Journal of Transatlantic Studies* 4, 2 (2014): 21–38, Webb, Jr. and Tamara Giles-Vernick, "Introduction," in *Global Health in Africa: Historical Perspectives on Disease*, ed. James L. A. Webb, Jr. and Tamara Giles-Vernick (Athens: Ohio University Press, 2013), 4, Steven Feierman and John Janzen, ed., *Health and Healing in Africa* (Berkeley: University of California Press, 1992), John Janzen, *The Quest for Therapy: Medical Pluralism in Lower Zaire* (Berkeley: University of California Press, 1978), Julie Livingston, *Debility and the Moral Imagination in Botswana* (Bloomington: Indiana University Press, 2005), Cristiana Bastos, "Medical Hybridisms and Social Boundaries: Aspects of Portuguese Colonialism in Africa and India in the Nineteenth Century," *Journal of Southern African Studies* 33, 4 (2007): 767, and Pier Larson, "'Capacities and Modes of Thinking': Intellectual Engagements and Subaltern Hegemony in the Early History of Malagasy Christianity," *American Historical Review* 102, 4 (October 1997): 969–1002.

[14]R. Menzies, I. Rocher, and B. Vissandjee, "Factors Associated with compliance in Treatment of Tuberculosis," *Tuberculosis and Lung Disease* 74 (1993): 36.

[15]Paul Farmer, *Infections and Inequalities: The Modern Plagues* (Berkeley, University of California Press, 1999), 225–227.

"everyday resistance" or reluctance to accept biomedical practices, akin to what James Scott has called "weapons of the weak."[16]

Building upon Paul Farmer's concept of structural inequality, Elisha Renne has emphasized the fact that effective public health compliance requires trust in government in her vivid comparison of polio eradication efforts in Northern Nigeria and Northeastern Ghana. She notes that Northern Nigerian parents' lack of faith in national health institutions and international public health organizations, inter-alia, contributes to low compliance with public health.[17] Yet this is not the case in Northeastern Ghana, where there is confidence in government and high rates of compliance and, as a result, fewer cases of polio than in Northern Nigeria. Renne points out that Northern Nigerian parents question why there is a focus on an apparently "minor" health problem because not many children get paralyzed by polio and because the government did not take polio to be an urgent health problem until the late 1950s and after independence.[18] They also ask why the government focuses exclusively on polio eradication while not providing basic primary health care for other diseases and why health personnel is taken away from basic primary health care to work on polio eradication initiatives. Northern Nigerian parents also question why the government does not provide polio immunizations with primary health care simultaneously instead of essentially placing the burden of basic health care on individuals and their families.[19]

Moreover what is striking about Northern Nigeria and Northeastern Ghana, as Renne points out, is that both are predominantly Muslim, largely agricultural, with high retentions of forms of "traditional organization," and both are in former British colonies and employ local medical practices, yet the responses to polio eradication initiatives could not have been more different.[20] In Ghana there was routine immunization and as a result there were no wild poliovirus infections between 2004 and 2007.[21]

[16] James Scott, *Weapons of the Weak: Everyday Forms of Peasant Resistance* (Yale University Press: New Haven, CT, 1985).

[17] Elisha P. Renne, *The Politics of Polio in Northern Nigeria* (Bloomington: Indiana University Press, 2010). On distrust of government in the era of Boko Haram, see Elisha P. Renne, "Parallel Dilemmas: Polio Transmission and Political Violence in Northern Nigeria," *Africa* 84, 3 (2014): 466–486.

[18] Renne, *The Politics of Polio*, 11, 24.

[19] Ibid., 14.

[20] Ibid., 87.

[21] Ibid., 86.

Renne adds that in Northeastern Ghana, although parents were aware of rumors about polio vaccine and infertility, just like in Northern Nigeria, these rumors were not widespread, and there was active participation of the Muslim community in polio eradication initiatives, with the immunization dates announced in mosques and immunizations carried out in Islamic schools. Renne concludes that the crucial distinguishing factor was the Ghanaian government's involvement in statewide primary health care programs, particularly routine immunizations, and its provision of basic health care infrastructure which bolstered public health cooperation with and even faith in government polio eradication efforts.[22]

This same scenario played out during the 2014–2015 West African Ebola Virus Disease pandemic which reinforced distrust of interventions by governments which only paid lip service to the provision of primary health care. The rumor that circulated in Sierra Leone that Ebola was not real and that it was just a trick used by doctors to steal people's blood was just one of the manifestations of this mistrust.[23] While some dismissed these stories as ridiculous conspiracy theories, others blamed the rapid spread of Ebola in West Africa on what they viewed as irrational beliefs and perilous cultural practices.[24] These include everything from the hunting and butchering of game or the so-called bushmeat, funeral practices in West African villages, to attributing Ebola sickness and mortality to witchcraft.[25]

[22] Ibid., 87–88.

[23] Shaunagh Connaire, "Ebola Outbreak" transcript, *PBS Frontline*, July 2014, http://www.pbs.org/wgbh/pages/frontline/health-science-technology/ebola-outbreak/transcript-67/ (24 December 2014). See also Jason Beaubien, "Rumor Patrol. No, A Snake In A Bag Did Not Cause Ebola," *NPR*, July 22, 2014, http://www.npr.org/blogs/goatsandsoda/2014/07/22/334022357/rumor-patrol-no-a-snake-in-a-bag-did-not-cause-ebola (24 December 2014).

[24] Mary Moran and Daniel Hoffman, "Ebola in Perspective," *Fieldsights – Hot Spots, Cultural Anthropology Online*, October 07, 2014, http://www.culanth.org/fieldsights/585-ebola-in-perspective (24 December 2014).

[25] Mike McGovern, "Bushmeat and the Politics of Disgust," *Fieldsights – Hot Spots, Cultural Anthropology Online*, October 07, 2014, http://www.culanth.org/fieldsights/588-bushmeat-and-the-politics-of-disgust (24 December 2014), Paul Richards and Alfred Mokuwa, "Village Funerals and the Spread of Ebola Virus Disease." *Fieldsights – Hot Spots, Cultural Anthropology Online*, October 07, 2014, http://www.culanth.org/fieldsights/590-village-funerals-and-the-spread-of-ebola-virus-disease (24 December 2014), and Catherine E. Bolten, "Articulating the Invisible: Ebola Beyond Witchcraft in Sierra Leone," *Fieldsights – Hot Spots, Cultural Anthropology Online*, October 07, 2014, http://www.culanth.org/

The legitimacy of the colonial state was thus central in determining African experiences with and responses to colonial public health.[26] Gloria Waite has shown that public health regulations existed in precolonial East-Central African societies and were not, therefore, newly introduced by Europeans in the twentieth century.[27] If public health encompasses all activities taken to improve a population's health, then rain-making and identification of sorcerers in precolonial Africa as well as control of infectious diseases, public sanitation works, and health education can be included.[28] Though contested, public health and control over healing in precolonial Africa were also central in gaining, maintaining, and exercising political power.[29] Thus when epidemics such as smallpox and other catastrophic events occurred, African authorities prohibited people from engaging in certain everyday activities, such as conjugal relationships as well as house-to-house visitations.[30] The contestation of public health

fieldsights/596-articulating-the-invisible-ebola-beyond-witchcraft-in-sierra-leone (24 December 2014).

[26] See also Jonathan Sadowsky, "The long Shadow of Colonialism: Why We Study Medicine in Africa," in *Medicine and Healing in Africa: Multidisciplinary Perspectives*, ed. Paula Viterbo and Kalala Ngalamulume (East Lansing: Michigan State University Press, 2010), p. 211 and Jonathan Sadowsky, *Imperial Bedlam*, 116.

[27] Gloria Waite, "Public Health in Pre-colonial East-Central Africa," in *The Social Basis of Health and Healing in Africa*, ed. Steven Feierman and John M. Janzen (Berkeley: University of California Press, 1992), 212–231.

[28] Ibid. See also Rebecca Marsland, "Who Are the 'Public' in Public Health?: Debating Crowds, Populations, and Publics in Tanzania," in *Making and Unmaking of Public Health in Africa: Ethnographic and Historical Perspectives*, ed. Ruth J. Prince and Rebecca Marsland (Athens: Ohio University Press, 2014), 75–95, Murray Last, "Understanding Health," in *Culture and Global Change*, ed. Tim Allen and Tracy Skelton, 72–86 (London: Routledge, 1999), Steven Feierman, "Colonizers, Scholars and the Creation of Invisible Histories," in *Beyond the Cultural Turn: New Directions in the Study of Society and Culture*, ed. Victoria E. Bonnell and Lynn Hunt, (Berkeley: University of California Press, 1999), 182–216; and Livingstone, *Debility and the Moral Imagination in Botswana*, 17.

[29] Prince, "Introduction: Situating Health and the Public in Africa," 16. See also Steven Feierman, "On Socially Composed Knowledge: Reconstructing a Shambaa Royal Ritual," in *In Search of A Nation: Histories of Authority and Dissidence in Tanzania*, ed. James L. Giblin and Gregory H. Maddox (Athens: Ohio University Press, 2005), 14–32.

[30] Ibid. The ruling elites included religious figures and chiefs who held power over land, its fertility, and its vitality through their persons, their use of medicines, and their control over ritual through their authority over healers and spirit mediums, rain-making, and witchcraft. With this power, they could cleanse the land and persons of pollution but could also limit growth and fertility. However, these elites could be deposed if they were unable or unwilling to respond to misfortune, and healers were not always close to those in political power; they

policy at the border thus reflected the questioning of colonial authority and contributed to reinforcing resistance to the most unpopular methods of biomedicine, hospitalization, and laboratory tests. This is evident in fears expressed in accounts of bodies disappearing in colonial hospitals never to be seen again, accounts of "blood sucking" for unknown reasons, and high death rates in hospitals contained in oral histories of colonial Africa.[31]

The Zimbabwe-Mozambique border was productive in the evolution and implementation of colonial public health policy. It was productive not only in breeding the obvious obstructions and frustrations but also in breeding desires and needs to cross it. The border produced opportunity as well as prohibition. This border-centric analysis calls into question the pervasive notion that cross-border movements pose health dangers, central to European settlers' claims of diffusion of disease, which influenced the evolution of colonial public health policy. Contrary to these claims, what largely affected disease ecologies were environmental and demographic changes engendered and perpetuated by colonialism, contributing to a worsening disease environment within the colonies. In fact, for many Africans, colonial restrictions on cross-border travel were harmful to African health because in precolonial times travel was a way of maintaining or regaining health, as in travel to see healers, obtain medicines and, especially in Shona society, travel to visit shrines of spirit mediums. As one village elder recalled, villagers sometimes crossed the border to visit African healers in Mozambique after being referred to them by Zimbabwean healers.[32] As Markku Hokkanen has shown in his work on the medical history of Malawi (Nyasaland), mobility, which was reflected in networks, was central part of "the intertwined medical cultures that shared the search for medicines in changing conditions."[33]

Not only did travel aid patients, but healers as well. Tracey Luedke and Harry West have convincingly argued in their edited volume exploring

could undermine such power or destabilize it. See also Feierman, "On Socially Composed Knowledge: Reconstructing a Shambaa Royal Ritual," 14–32.

[31] These fears were not confined to Southern Africa. They were present in many African societies. For East Africa, see Ndege, *Health, State, and Society in Kenya*, 6 and Luise White, *Speaking with Vampires: Rumor and History in Colonial Africa* (Berkeley: University of California Press, 2000), 89.

[32] Interview, Vheremu, Zimbabwe, December 24, 2016.

[33] Markku Hokkanen, *Medicine, Mobility and the Empire: Nyasaland Networks, 1859–1960* (Manchester: Manchester University Press, 2017), 2.

large-scale circulation and the accompanying border-crossing of "people and spirits, objects and substances, practices and techniques, discourses, ideas, and memories associated with healing in southeast Africa" that border crossings empowered healers and made their work of healing possible.[34]

Therefore, in spite of twentieth-century hopes that globalization would usher in a borderless and deterritorialized world, Yakubu Joseph and Rainer Rothfuss note that borders have remained an integral part of human political and social life and are even adapting to evolving spatio-temporal conditions.[35] They also observe that interdisciplinary border research has witnessed a paradigm shift from a state-centric national security focus to a decentralized human security concern, where the state and the population are all active players and shapers of borders. Hence, the study of borders has moved from the concept of "space- and time-oriented fixed demarcating lines" to bordering, with "an emphasis on the symbolic and social practices of spatial differentiation aimed at controlling movement of people both into and within a securitized space."[36]

There is a considerable amount of literature on African borders and borderlands, particularly in analyses of African experiences of colonialism, labor migration, economic transformation, as well as resistance to colonial rule.[37] Some scholars consider borders as permeable, arguing that have shown that border zones are "shadowy places," often sites of activities such as smuggling, local "vigilante" justice, and unauthorized movements that are "officially illegal but have become accepted features of everyday life for resident populations."[38] This is in line with a recent reconsideration

[34] See Luedke and West, "Healing Divides," 3–4.

[35] Yakubu Joseph and Rainer Rothfuss, "Symbolic Bordering and the Securitization of Identity Markers in Nigeria's Ethno-Religiously Segregated City of Jos," in Reece Jones and Corey Johnson (eds), *Placing the Border in Everyday Life* (Surrey: Ashgate, 2014): 167.

[36] Ibid. See also Ronen Shamir, "Without Borders? Notes on Globalization as a Mobility Regime," *Sociological Theory* 23, 2 (2005): 200.

[37] See, for example, S. Berry, "Crossing boundaries, Debating African Studies," Paper presented at the Fifth Annual Penn African Studies Workshop (October 17, 1997), available at http://www.africa.upenn.edu/Workshop/sara.html, retrieved on 20 August 2013, Eric Allina-Pisano, "Borderlands, Boundaries, and the Contours of Colonial Rule," Patrick Harries, *Work, Culture, and Identity: Migrant Laborers in Mozambique and South Africa, c. 1860–1910* (Portsmouth, Heinemann, 1994), A. I. Asiwaju, "Migrations as Revolt: The Example of the Ivory Coast and Upper Volta before 1945," *Journal of African History*, 17, 4 (1976), pp. 577–594.

[38] Maxim Bolt, "Waged Entrepreneurs, Policed Informality: Work, the Regulation of Space and the Economy of the Zimbabwean–South African Border," *Africa*, 82, 1 (2012), p. 112.

of the idea of "arbitrary" borders in Africa to highlight the fact that borders were also zones of opportunity and that most of them are "naturalized" today and not contested as such by African actors.[39] Other scholars, however, say that borders are powerful, arguing that fixed territorial boundaries often operate to restrict people's movements and limit people's access to opportunities and resources.[40]

In Southern Africa, the presence of the Zimbabwe-Mozambique border meant that, while the intrusive colonial public health measures were constant and pervasive, they were not always effective. The Zimbabwe-Mozambique border region constitutes an area whose epidemiology was fundamentally affected by cross-border movements. In a region where the

See also, van Schendel, W, "Spaces of Engagement: How Borderlands, Illegal Flows and Territorial States Interlock," in I. Abraham and W. van Schendel (eds), *Illicit Flows and Criminal Things: States, Borders, and the Other Side of Globalization* (Bloomington IN, Indiana University Press, 2005), pp. 38–68, H. Cunningham and J. Heyman, "Introduction: Mobilities and Enclosures at Borders," *Identities* 11, 2 (2004): 289–302, and Blair Rutherford, "The Politics of Boundaries: The Shifting Terrain of Belonging for Zimbabweans in a South African Border Zone," *African Diaspora: Transnational Journal of Culture, Economy & Society* 4, 2 (2011): 207–229.

[39] Allina-Pisano, "Borderlands, Boundaries, and the Contours of Colonial rule," p. 60. See also Eric Allina-Pisano, "Negotiating Colonialism: Africans, the State, and the Market in Manica District, Mozambique, 1895–c. 1935" (PhD thesis, Yale University, 2002) and Eric Allina, *Slavery By Any Other Name: African Life Under Company Rule in Colonial Mozambique* (Charlottesville: University of Virginia Press, 2012). See also Ana Cristina Roque, "A History of Mozambique's Southern Border: The Archives of the Portuguese Commission of Cartography," in Steven Van Wolputte (ed.) *Borderlands and Frontiers in Africa* (Berlin: LIT VERLAG Dr. W. Hopf, 2013), 23–54, Dereje Feyissa and Markus Virgil Hoehne, "State Borders and Borderlands as Resources," in Dereje Feyissa and Markus Virgil Hoehne (eds.) *Borders and Borderlands as Resources in the Horn of Africa* (Suffolk: James Currey, 2010), p. 1–7, Steven Van Wolputte, "Introduction: Living the Border," in Steven Van Wolputte (ed.) *Borderlands and Frontiers in Africa* (Berlin: LIT VERLAG Dr. W. Hopf, 2013), 2, V. Das and D. Poole, "State and its Margins: Comparative ethnographies," in V. Das and D. Poole (eds) *Anthropology in the Margins of the State* (New Delhi: Oxford University Press, 2004), 3–33, Ana L. Tsing, "From the margins," *Cultural Anthropology* 9, 3 (1994): 279–297, Benedikt Korff and Timothy Raeymaekers, "Introduction: Border, Frontier and the Geography of Rule at the Margins of the State," in Benedikt Korff and Timothy Raemaekers (eds.) *Violence on the Margins: States, Conflict, and Borderlands* (New York: Palgrave Macmillan, 2013), 4, and Karen Büscher and Gillian Mathys, "Navigating the Urban 'In-Between Space': Local Livelihood and Identity Strategies in Exploiting the Goma/Gisenyi Border," in Benedikt Korff and Timothy Raemaekers (eds.) *Violence on the Margins: States, Conflict, and Borderlands* (New York: Palgrave Macmillan, 2013), 120.

[40] See, for example, A. I. Asiwaju (ed.), *Partitioned Africans: Ethnic Relations Across Africa's International Boundaries, 1884–1984* (New York, St. Martins, 1985).

population was highly mobile, public health policies restricted to territorial boundaries encountered enormous difficulties in addressing infectious and communicable diseases, such as smallpox, sleeping sickness, and sexually transmitted diseases (STDs) such as syphilis.[41] Therefore, while the border was permeable, it still played a crucial role in the evolution of colonial public health services. It was this conditional permeability of the border which made it so powerful, prompting colonial authorities who were fearful of the spread of infections to act.[42]

Yet the Zimbabwe-Mozambique border was still difficult and constraining because although people crossed it, they lost some of the rights and securities they enjoyed at home.[43] This conditional permeability of border characterized much of Southern Africa, demonstrating that colonial powers drew Africa's borders as "sifters of labour rather than as barriers to its movement."[44] The border was also a zone of opportunity, with African mobility in the borderland serving a powerful force in the constitution of colonial power.[45] For instance, African chiefs in Mozambique used the border as a powerful negotiating tool with colonial administrators to avoid labor conscription by the Mozambique Company government. Thus, while the Zimbabwe-Mozambique border was permeable and contested, it was still powerful in shaping the course of events because this permeability of the border prompted colonial authorities to act in order to restrict movements of Africans and their livestock.

[41] See also James L. A. Webb, Jr., "The First Large-Scale Use of Synthetic Insecticide for Malaria Control in Tropical Africa: Lessons from Liberia, 1945–62," in *Global Health in Africa: Historical Perspectives on Disease*, ed. James L. A. Webb, Jr. and Tamara Giles-Vernick (Athens: Ohio University Press, 2013), 12. This is similar to what the British experienced in the Anglo-Egyptian Sudan, where medical and administrative personnel faced the contradiction of public health's need for impermeable borders in contrast to the socio-economic need for permeable ones, see Heather Bell, *Frontiers of Medicine in the Anglo-Egyptian Sudan, 1899–1940* (Oxford: Clarendon Press, 1999), 10.

[42] See also Francis Dube, "'In the Border Regions.'"

[43] David Hughes, *From Enslavement to Environmentalism: Politics on a Southern African Frontier* (Seattle, University of Washington Press, 2006), 76.

[44] Ibid., 76–77.

[45] Allina-Pisano, 'Borderlands, Boundaries, and the Contours of Colonial rule', 60. See also Allina-Pisano, "Negotiating Colonialism," and Allina, *Slavery By Any Other Name*. See also Roque, "A History of Mozambique's Southern Border," Feyissa and Hoehne, "State Borders and Borderlands as Resources," 1–7, Van Wolputte, "Introduction: Living the Border," 2, Das and Poole, "State and its Margins," 3–33, Tsing, "From the margins," Korff and Raeymaekers, "Introduction," 4, and Büscher and Mathys, "Navigating the Urban 'In-Between Space.'" 120.

This border was therefore both restrictive and porous at the same time. It was restrictive because colonial officials monitored and limited movements of people and livestock across it. This often happened on official ports of entry which were easily accessible, usually by road and on foot. While these official ports of entry regulated movement, there were numerous paths that Africans used to cross the border, where nobody could restrict them. This demonstrates that the border was porous. However, these paths had restrictions of a different nature. They were not easily accessible. They usually were in areas of difficult and hazardous terrain, such as mountains. Africans therefore had to climb up and down steep mountains, usually with heavy luggage. These restrictions thus caused much hardship to villagers and to women, the elderly, and children in particular, who, in the absence of colonial health services in the rural areas were left with few alternatives. For the majority of African men recruited to work on government and white settler projects, at least, there was a semblance of health care provided, albeit only to keep the labor force healthy and maintain or increase productivity.

While many studies have focused on migration in Southern Africa, few have attempted to analyze migration in light of disease and public health although there is growing interest in new ways of understanding migration, ecology, disease, health, and colonialism. Also, while there are important studies addressing various aspects of medicine and health in Africa such as the various African responses to Western medicine, including resistance, acceptance, and adaptation to African conditions,[46] the role of intermediaries and subordinates in public health,[47] the public health consequences of the gap between the biomedical and social sciences,[48] and the

[46] See, for example, David Baronov, *The African Transformation of Western Medicine and the Dynamics of Global Cultural Exchange* (Philadelphia: Temple University Press, 2008), Ndege, *Health, State, and Society in Kenya*, Tracy J. Luedke and Harry G. West, "Healing Divides," 4. See also Comaroff and Comaroff, *Of Revelation and Revolution. Volume Two*, 364, Adam Mohr "Missionary Medicine and Akan Therapeutics: Illness, Health and Healing in Southern Ghana's Basel Mission, 1828–1918," *Journal of Religion in Africa* 39 (2009): 437, Steven Feierman and John Janzen, ed., *Health and Healing in Africa* (Berkeley: University of California Press, 1992), Janzen, *The Quest for Therapy*, Julie Livingston, *Debility and the Moral Imagination in Botswana*, Bastos, "Medical Hybridisms and Social Boundaries," 767, and Larson, "'Capacities and Modes of Thinking,'" 4.

[47] Ryan Johnson and Khalid Amna (eds.), *Public Health in the British Empire: Intermediaries, Subordinates, and the Practice of Public Health, 1850–1960* (New York: Routledge, 2012).

[48] James L. A. Webb, Jr. and Tamara Giles-Vernick, ed., *Global Health in Africa: Historical Perspectives on Disease* (Athens: Ohio University Press, 2013).

meaning of public health in Africa,[49] to date, not much has been done to examine the relationship between borders and health in the African context. Nevertheless, there has been recent and considerable interest in studies conceived at the scale of not one colony or one empire but rather focused on intercolonial and inter-imperial circulations, exchanges, and boundaries.[50]

Existing works on borders and health examine cooperation largely from the metropolitan level, looking at the training of practitioners and testing of drugs, and do not specifically deal with the implications borders on public health.[51] Allison Bashford has noted that the desire to combat infectious disease has been an arm of geopolitics and disease management, with quarantine lines in Africa serving as boundary lines for new "international" borders between Sudan and Egypt, between Uganda, French Congo, and Belgian Congo.[52] Along the same lines, Heather Bell has written about the role of colonial medicine in the establishment of colonies, the protection of a profession, and the control of disease through the demarcation of borders.[53]

In Mozambique and Zimbabwe, the border provided both opportunity and prohibition, inspiring some distrust of public health in spite of claims that colonial medicine broke down the African distrust of European medicine.[54] The architects of colonial rule had placed much hope in the cultural power of colonial medicine. They hoped that colonial medicine's perceived

[49] Ruth J. Prince and Rebecca Marsland, ed., *Making and Unmaking of Public Health in Africa: Ethnographic and Historical Perspectives* (Athens: Ohio University Press, 2014).

[50] See, for example, Anne Digby, Waltraud Ernst, and Projit B. Mukharji, ed., *Crossing Colonial Historiographies: Histories of Colonial and Indigenous Medicines in Transnational Perspective* (Cambridge: Cambridge Scholars Publishing, 2010), Frederick Cooper and Ann Stoler, ed., *Tensions of Empire: Colonial Cultures in A Bourgeois World* (Berkeley: University of California Press, 1997), Warwick Anderson, *Colonial Pathologies: American Tropical Medicine, Race, and Hygiene in the Philippines* (Durham: Duke University Press, 2006), Deborah J. Neill, *Networks in Tropical Medicine: Internationalism, Colonialism, and the Rise of a Medical Specialty, 1890–1930* (Stanford: Stanford University Press, 2012), and Alison Bashford, ed., *Medicine at the Border: Disease, Globalization and Security, 1850 to the Present* (New York: Palgrave Macmillan, 2006).

[51] See, for example, Neill, *Networks in Tropical Medicine.*

[52] Alison Bashford, "'The Age of Universal Contagion': History, Disease and Globalization," in Alison Bashford, ed., *Medicine at the Border: Disease, Globalization and Security, 1850 to the Present* (New York: Palgrave Macmillan, 2006), 2. See Bell, *Frontiers of Medicine*, 4.

[53] Bell, *Frontiers of Medicine*, 233.

[54] D. M. Blair, Foreword to *A Service to the Sick: A History of the Health Services for Africans in Southern Rhodesia, 1890–1953* (Gwelo: Mambo Press, 1976), 6–8.

efficacy would convince colonial subjects to accept imperial rule. They were also convinced that colonial medicine would facilitate the creation of a new cosmology by eroding the influence of indigenous belief systems, thereby easing the development of colonial, capitalist social forms.[55] Some even went as far as exploring the potential usefulness of Western biomedicine as a tool of governance. The French in colonial Cameroon, for example, made an unsuccessful attempt to hand over the political reins to doctors under a utopia of "medical governance" between 1939 and 1948.[56] However, these grandiose aims of colonial authorities have been called into question by studies showing the limits of both hegemonic power and hegemonic desires of colonial medical institutions.[57]

Western European ideas of public health achieved limited success because they lacked resonance with African socio-economic and political conditions and prevailing systems of health management.[58] Even with the best intentions, colonial authorities faced unintended consequences and dilemmas. If they did not intervene in medical emergencies they would be accused of nonchalance to the plight of colonial subjects, but if they intervened with vigor they were often accused of neglecting social and economic circumstances.[59] However, African resentment was also tied to the growth of colonial discrimination against Africans and African doctors, even those with biomedical training.[60] Hence, as global public health initiatives rooted in Western biomedicine attempt to cross the hurdle of earned distrust, "the historical significance of colonial medicine may lie

[55] Jonathan Sadowsky, *Imperial Bedlam*, 116. See, for example, David Arnold. *Colonizing the Body: State Medicine and Epidemic Disease in Nineteenth-Century India* (Berkeley: University of California Press, 1993), David Arnold, "Introduction: Disease, Medicine and Empire," in *Imperial Medicine and Indigenous Societies*, ed. David Arnold (Manchester: Manchester University Press, 1988), 16, and John Comaroff and Jean Comaroff, *Of revelation and revolution: Christianity, colonialism, and consciousness in South Africa* (Chicago: University of Chicago Press, 1991), and Francis Dube, "Medicine without Borders."

[56] Guillaume Lachenal, "Experimental Hubris and Medical Powerlessness: Notes from a Colonial Utopia, Cameroon, 1939–1949," in *Rethinking Biomedicine and Governance in Africa: Contributions from Anthropology*, ed. Paul Wenzel Geissler, Richard Rottenburg, and Julia Zenker (Bielefeld: Verlag, 2012), 119.

[57] Ibid. See also Meghan Vaughan, "Healing and Curing Issues in the Social History and Anthropology of Medicine in Africa," *Social History of Medicine* 7, 2 (1994): 288.

[58] Lyons, "Public Health in Colonial Africa," 356.

[59] Myron Echenberg, *Black Death, White Medicine: Bubonic Plague and the Politics of Public Health in Colonial Senegal, 1914–1945* (Portsmouth, NH: Heinemann, 2002), 4.

[60] Sadowsky, "The long Shadow of Colonialism," 210. See also Adell Patton, Jr., *Physicians, Colonial Racism, and Diaspora in West Africa* (Gainesville: University of Florida, 1996).

less in its intention or ability to colonize the mind than in its tendency more simply to control or neglect the ailing person."[61]

Reflecting the dynamism of African societies, however, while the Shona of the Zimbabwe-Mozambique border region tended to dislike intrusive and discriminatory preventative public health policies, they were willing to experiment with new ideas, particularly out-patient treatment services. Thus, as Africans critiqued certain aspects of Western biomedicine, there were accommodations and compromises.[62] They were discouraged, however, by the failure of colonial governments to provide adequate treatment-based services for Africans. This attitude of colonial governments toward Africans only served to prove that the provision of health services for Africans was driven by European fears of infection and economic imperatives rather than the concern for Africans. The failure to establish comprehensive and effective treatment services diminished the success of public health programs. Hence, contrary to popular belief, Africans were not distrustful of Western medicine *per se*; they were distrustful of the methods of delivery and what those methods represented, everything from racism and coercion to paternalism and control.

In the Zimbabwe-Mozambique border region, European settler fears of infection were a major impetus for public health measures as Europeans considered Africans to be a source of a myriad of infectious and communicable diseases.[63] Thus disease was a powerful element in European perceptions of indigenous society because it cultivated Europeans' growing sense of their inherent racial and physical supremacy.[64] These fears of infection account for the differences in the degree of implementation of public health measures between Mozambique, which had a small European settler population, and Zimbabwe, which had a considerable European settler population on estates, on farms, and in towns. The Zimbabwean side consequently developed a more rigorous approach to public health than Mozambique due to the pressure from the settler population. However, most of these settlers' fears stemmed from misunderstandings of epidemiology and were often grossly exaggerated as well as bluntly racist in nature. Yet, regardless of whether these theories were accurate or not, the policies that emerged from them adversely affected the Shona people. For

[61] Sadowsky, *Imperial Bedlam*, 116.
[62] Ndege, *Health, State, and Society in Kenya*, 2.
[63] Achola, "The Public Health Ordinance Policy," 114–115.
[64] Arnold, "Introduction," 7–8.

example, some Mozambican migrant workers were afraid that their distinctive smallpox vaccination scars would make them easily identifiable for deportation while seeking work in South Africa.

Although colonial powers attempted to use medicine as a "tool" of empire and as "biopower" to soften the coercive features of colonial rule by developing a broader imperial dominance than could be acquired by subjugation alone,[65] they failed in this respect. For in spite of the Enlightenment ideal of implementing biomedicine impartially, colonial biomedicine was full of internal contradictions and external dissensions.[66] Racial and colonial stereotypes, the denigration of Africans and Africa, blood theft rumors, misunderstandings, violence, and repression that took place around biomedical practice all emphasize that biomedicine was unpredictable and incoherent.[67]

An analysis of the development of colonial health services in Africa shows that although each European nation intervened in varied ways, in general the French, Portuguese, Belgian, and the British developed medical services that depended heavily on technology and ignored social and economic circumstances.[68] From the late nineteenth century to the 1920s

[65] Ibid., 16. See also Martin Shapiro, "Medicine in the service of colonialism: medical care in Portuguese Africa, 1885–1974" (Ph.D. dissertation, University of California, Los Angeles, 1983), Roy MacLeod, preface to *Disease, Medicine, Empire: Perspectives on Western Medicine and the Experience of European Expansion* (New York: Routledge, 1988), x and Spencer H. Brown, "A Tool of Empire: The British Medical Establishment in Lagos, 1861–1905," *International Journal of African Historical Studies* 37, 2 (2004): 309.

[66] Poonam Bala and Amy Kaler, "Introduction: Contested 'Ventures': Explaining Biomedicine in Colonial Contexts," in *Biomedicine as a Contested Site: Some Revelations in Imperial Contexts*, ed. Poonam Bala (Lanham, MD: Lexington Books, 2009), 3.

[67] Prince, "Introduction: Situating Health and the Public in Africa," 13. See also White, *Speaking with Vampires*, Nancy Rose Hunt, *A Colonial Lexicon: Of Birth Ritual, Medicalization, and Mobility in the Congo* (Durham: Duke University Press, 1999), Steven Feierman, "Colonizers, Scholars and the Creation of Invisible Histories," in *Beyond the Cultural Turn: New Directions in the Study of Society and Culture*, ed. Victoria E. Bonnell and Lynn Hunt (Berkeley: University of California Press, 1999), 182–216.

[68] Randall Packard, "Visions of Postwar Health and Development and Their Impact on Public Health Interventions in the Developing World," in *Internal Development and the Social Sciences: Essays on the History and Politics of Knowledge*, ed. Fredrick Cooper and Randall Packard (Berkeley: University of California Press, 1997), 95. See also Megan Vaughan, *Curing Their Ills: Colonial Power and African Illness.* (Stanford: Stanford University Press, 1993), Michael Worboys, "The Emergence of Tropical Medicine," in *Perspectives on the Emergence of Scientific Disciplines*, ed. Gerald Lemaine, et al. (The Hague: Mouton, 1976), 75–98, Michael Worboys, "The Discovery of Colonial Malnutrition between the Wars," in *Imperial Medicine and Indigenous Societies*, ed. David Arnold

colonial authorities focused their efforts on improving the health of European settlers and in controlling epidemics of infectious and tropical diseases that threatened the supply and efficiency of African labor.[69] Wherever disease was believed to threaten the health of the African labor force, for example, in towns and mining centers, colonial governments established health services for Africans in the early years of colonial rule. For rural Africans, however, the encounter with Western biomedicine during this period was mostly limited to intrusive public health campaigns against diseases such as sleeping sickness, plague, and smallpox, and Christian medical services such as those of the American Board of Commissioners for Foreign Missions (ABCFM, hereafter American Board Mission) in the Zimbabwe-Mozambique border region. There is no doubt that financial constraints played a significant part in this lop-sided development of health services, but this should also be viewed more in terms of colonial priorities than simply the lack of funds. These priorities that placed emphasis on European health and economic well-being dictated where the available resources were spent, and it was not on African health *per se*. The early coercive and violent campaigns, however, did much to shape African attitudes toward Western biomedicine.[70] Later in the 1930s and 1940s, there were limited attempts to extend health services to Africans in rural areas.[71] For colonial Zimbabwe and Mozambique, concerns about settler health were still paramount and investment in African health was not an end in itself, but was meant to benefit white settlers and colonial economies.

The writing of the history of colonial public health has moved from celebratory accounts of colonial medical services and "heroic" medical

(Manchester: Manchester University Press, 1988), 208–223, John Farley, *Bilharzia: A History of Imperial Tropical Medicine*, (Cambridge: Cambridge University Press, 1991), L. Doyal, *The Political Economy of Health* (London: Pluto Press, 1979), and James L. A. Webb, Jr. and Tamara Giles-Vernick, "Introduction," 1–2. See also W. Penn Handwerker, Foreword to *Indigenous Theories of Contagious Disease* (Walnut Creek, CA: AltaMira Press, 1999), 7.

[69] Prince, "Introduction: Situating Health and the Public in Africa," 17. See also Packard, "Visions of Postwar Health and Development," 93–115 and Michael Gelfand, *A Service to the Sick: A History of the Health Services for Africans in Southern Rhodesia, 1890–1953* (Gwelo: Mambo Press, 1976), 40.

[70] See, for example, Vaughan, *Curing Their Ills* and White, *Speaking with Vampires*.

[71] Packard, "Visions of Postwar Health and Development," 93–115.

men, particularly in British colonies,[72] to the political ecology of disease scholars of the 1970s who challenged this perception. These scholars contended that political, economic, and social transformations brought about by colonization had disrupted existing ecological relationships and the health of local populations.[73] The results of these environmental changes were epidemic outbreaks which increased the burden of disease in colonies especially on vulnerable sections of society such as women, children, and rural inhabitants.[74] The failure of colonial public health to convince Africans of the efficacy of Western biomedicine has also led to the questioning of the image of an omnipotent colonial state.[75] There has also been an effort to focus on subordinate and intermediary agents who formed the backbone of colonial medical services, instead of merely focusing on administrators.[76] In the same vein, new literature on colonial European and indigenous nurses has examined their role as intermediaries and "cultural brokers."[77] These works reflect new trends in historiography that situate colonial health and medicine within broader international, global, and transnational contexts.[78] This approach is credited with breaking down the notion that indigenous healing was traditional and unchanging while Western medicine was dynamic and modern.[79]

[72] See, for example, Gelfand, *A Service to the Sick* and Michael Gelfand, *Proud Record in Health Services in Rhodesia and Nyasaland*. Salisbury, Southern Rhodesia, 1959.

[73] See John Ford. *The Role of the Trypanosomiases in African Ecology: a Study of the Tsetse Fly Problem* (Oxford: Clarendon Press, 1971).

[74] Feierman, "Struggles for Control," 12.

[75] See, for example, Mark Harrison, *Public Health in British India: Anglo-Indian Preventive Medicine, 1859–1914* (Cambridge: Cambridge University Press, 1994).

[76] Ryan Johnson and Amna Khalid, "Introduction," in *Public Health in the British Empire: Intermediaries, Subordinates, and the Practice of Public Health, 1850–1960*, ed. Ryan Johnson and Amna Khalid (Routledge: New York, 2012), 2.

[77] See, for example, Anne Digby and Helen Sweet, "Nurses as Cultural Brokers in Twentieth-Century South Africa," in *Plural Medicine, Tradition and Modernity, 1800–2000*, ed. Waltraud Ernst (London: Routledge, 2002), 113–129.

[78] See, for example, Anne Digby, Waltraud Ernst, and Projit B. Mukharji, ed., *Crossing Colonial Historiographies*.

[79] Johnson and Khalid, "Introduction," 12. See also, Waltraud Ernst, ed., *Plural Medicine, Tradition and Modernity, 1800–2000* (London: Routledge, 2002) and Karen Flint, *Healing Traditions: African Medicine, Cultural Exchange, and Competition in South Africa, 1820–1948* (Athens: Ohio University Press, 2008).

Overview

Public Health at the Border is divided into three parts: "Life and Health Before the Border," "Life and Health with the Border," and "The Border and Public Health." In Part I, Chap. 2 discusses the landscape, geography, and disease environment of the Zimbabwe-Mozambique border region. It provides a vivid sense of the environmental diversity to show why it was important for people to access resources that lay across the border. The reason for this was that the organization of precolonial public health largely overlapped with environmental differences, with people in semi-arid areas concerned about rainfall, for example. Chapter 2 also details the social, political, and economic forces that determined patterns of mobility before the colonization of the region in 1890. These forces included trade and exchange, kinship or family connections, hunting, herding, and traveling for health reasons.

Part II then deals with the imposition of the border and the creation of a public health problem from 1890. Here, Chap. 3 details the process of colonization, the demarcation of the border, and subsequent border restrictions as well as the establishment of Christian mission stations which played a crucial role in the provision of health services for the Shona people of the border region. Chapter 4 then examines the general oppression that followed the establishment of colonial rule, with an emphasis on land alienation, taxation, forced labor, and dipping fees, among other things, arguing that these, together with border restrictions, contributed to the contestations of the border and colonial authority. It shows how the conjunction of a particular colonized society, a distinctive kind of colonialism and a particular territorial border, generated forms of low compliance with public health.

The implications of the border for the control of infectious diseases such as trypanosomiasis, syphilis, and smallpox as well as the provision of health services for Africans are taken up in Part III. Thus, Part III examines colonial public health efforts and African evasion of cross-border restrictions and other forms of noncompliance. It shows that low compliance with public health resulted from a lack of trust and fear of government institutions, as well as the discriminatory application of public health. Hence, Chap. 5 deals with the increased incidence of sleeping sickness (trypanosomiasis) as a result of environmental changes engendered by the imposition of colonial rule. The attempt to control sleeping sickness contributed to colonial efforts to restrict the mobility of African cattle herders across the border, particularly after 1900 as the much hoped for gold wealth did not materialize and the colonial states emphasized agriculture and cattle ranching as the mainstays of the economy.

The war on epidemics such as smallpox is the subject of Chap. 6, which examines smallpox epidemics and control, whose incidence also increased as a result of the establishment of colonial rule in 1890. It shows how the border continued to be an obstacle to the implementation of effective regional public health policy. The wide-ranging impact of colonial public health is taken up in this chapter as well. This chapter argues that in their attempts to monitor the border for public health purposes, colonial governments went as far as depriving Africans of their right to congregate for religious purposes beginning in the 1920s. For some members of African Independent Churches, therefore, colonial interference with faith healing became one of the most important grievances against colonial rule.

Chapter 7 then examines the implications of the border on the control of STDs, particularly syphilis. It argues that as a result of the growth of agriculture, cattle ranching, mining, and urbanization from the 1920s, all of which depended largely on African male labor, the incidence of STDs increased in mining and farming compounds and urban areas, particularly in Zimbabwe. Thus, beginning in the 1920s, in an effort to control STDs and to regulate African mobility, colonial officials compelled Shona men and women to undergo shameful "medical examinations" which interfered with Shona's ideas of privacy and masculinity.

The extension of curative health services, through hospitals and clinics, to rural Africans is the subject of Chap. 8. Chapter 8 considers the spatial distribution of health services based on borders, both internal and intercolonial. It continues the theme of the fear of diffusion of disease and its impact on public health. The borders included rural/urban, African/European, and Zimbabwe/Mozambique. This chapter contends that treating disease in rural Africans was the European settlers' last line of defense against disease, which partially explains why efforts to expand the services came relatively late in the 1930s and early 1940s and also why they were influenced by the size and political clout of European settlers in each colony. This chapter therefore argues that while the Shona people of the border region were open to innovation, they were discouraged by the discriminatory nature and inadequacy of colonial medical services. It clearly contrasts low compliance with public health and willingness to benefit from curative biomedicine, which did not require the same trust in government. Parts II and III thus examine border restrictions imposed by the colonial governments, how these restrictions changed over time, and how and why villagers and townsfolk evaded these restrictions on cross-border movement. The Conclusion, which is Chap. 9, then considers the significance of all these developments.

The research for *Public Health at the Border* occurred between 2003 and 2010 in both Zimbabwe and Mozambique. Sources include documents from the National Archives of Zimbabwe in Harare (formerly Salisbury) and the documents of the Companhia de Moçambique (hereafter Mozambique Company) from Arquivo Histórico de Moçambique in Maputo, largely comprising reports and correspondence. The Mozambique Company governed central Mozambique for 50 years, from 1892 to 1942, and left much documentation that deals with many aspects of its reign, including health issues. After 1942, the sources on the Mozambican section of the border region become rare. That is where oral histories come in. In general, the sources for Zimbabwe are more readily accessible than those for Mozambique.

In addition to archival documents, this book also made use of materials from the Departments of Agriculture and Natural Resources in Zimbabwe and the Direcção Nacional de Pecuária and the Department of Tsetse Control in Mozambique. The records of the American Board of Commissioners for Foreign Missions, housed in the Houghton Library of Harvard University in Boston, Massachusetts, the United States, are also pivotal in this research. The missionary sources consist mainly of correspondence between missionaries abroad and the directors of the American Board of Commissioners for Foreign Missions in Boston and reports on the medical, evangelistic, and educational activities of the missionaries. These records also include reports on the relations between the mission and colonial governments and minutes of meetings.

Oral histories also play an important role, particularly in determining African perceptions of disease and healing, as well as the impact of colonial public health policy. These were collected between 2006 and 2007, some by the author and others by research assistants. The interviews were conducted in Shona, a language spoken on both sides of the Zimbabwe-Mozambique border. The places visited on the Zimbabwean side include Penhalonga (Tsvingwe Village, Old West Mine Compound, Elim Mission), Zimunya (Chitakatira, Mvududu, Nehwangura, and Nyamakamba villages), Ngaone, and in areas surrounding Mt. Selinda (Chirinda), such as Beacon Hill, Days Hill, Holland Farm, Maengeni Village, and Vheremu. A few more interviews were conducted at Tanganda Halt in the semi-arid part of Chipinge district and in Harare. On the Mozambican side, interviews were carried out in Chambuta and Zangiro in the Sussundenga district, and at Spungabera and areas surrounding it, such as Mamuse, Makubvu, Mpanyeya, and Muedzwa in Mossurize district. The names of some interviewees have been intentionally left out because most of the interviews were conducted with the understanding that the names would not be made public due to political considerations. When these interviews were collected, some interviewees in the border region were afraid of being accused of talking to foreign media and being "sellouts" due to the political situation in Zimbabwe at that time.

References

Achola, Milcah Amolo. "The Public Health Ordinance Policy of the Nairobi Municipal/City Council 1945–62." In *African Historians and African Voices: Essays presented of Professor Bothwell Allan Ogot*, edited by E. S. Atieno Odhiambo. Basel: P. Schlettwein Publishing, 2001.

Allina-Pisano, Eric. "Negotiating Colonialism: Africans, the State, and the Market in Manica District, Mozambique, 1895–c. 1935." PhD Dissertation, Yale University, May 2002.

———. "Borderlands, Boundaries, and the Contours of Colonial Rule: African Labour in Manica District, Mozambique, c. 1904–1908." *International Journal of African Historical Studies*, 36, 1 (2003): 59–82.

Allina, Eric. *Slavery By Any Other Name: African Life Under Company Rule in Colonial Mozambique.* Charlottesville: University of Virginia Press, 2012.

Arnold, David. "Introduction: disease, medicine and empire." In *Imperial Medicine and Indigenous Societies*, edited by David Arnold. 1–26. Manchester: Manchester University Press, 1988.

———. *Colonizing the Body: State Medicine and Epidemic Disease in nineteenth-century India.* Berkeley: University of California Press, 1993.

Asiwaju, A. I. "Migrations as Revolt: The Example of the Ivory Coast and Upper Volta before 1945." *Journal of African History*, 17, 4 (1976): 577–594.

———. ed. *Partitioned Africans: Ethnic Relations Across Africa's International Boundaries, 1884–1984.* New York, St. Martins, 1985.

Bala, Poonam and Kaler, Amy. "Introduction: Contested 'Ventures': Explaining Biomedicine in Colonial Contexts." In *Biomedicine as a Contested Site: Some Revelations in Imperial Contexts*, edited by Poonam Bala. 1–7. Lanham, MD: Lexington Books, 2009.

Bashford, Alison. "'The Age of Universal Contagion': History, Disease and Globalization." In *Medicine at the Border: Disease, Globalization and Security,*

1850 to the Present, edited by Alison Bashford. 1–17. New York: Palgrave Macmillan, 2006.

Bolten, Catherine E. "Articulating the Invisible: Ebola Beyond Witchcraft in Sierra Leone." *Fieldsights – Hot Spots, Cultural Anthropology Online*, October 07, 2014. http://www.culanth.org/fieldsights/596-articulating-the-invisible-ebola-beyond-witchcraft-in-sierra-leone (24 December 2014).

Baronov, David. *The African Transformation of Western Medicine and the Dynamics of Global Cultural Exchange*. Philadelphia: Temple University Press, 2008.

Bastos, Cristiana. "Medical Hybridisms and Social Boundaries: Aspects of Portuguese Colonialism in Africa and India in the Nineteenth Century." *Journal of Southern African Studies* 33, no. 4 (2007): 767–782.

Bell, Heather. *Frontiers of Medicine in the Anglo-Egyptian Sudan, 1899–1940*. Oxford: Clarendon Press, 1999.

Berry, S. 'Crossing boundaries, Debating African Studies', Paper presented at the Fifth Annual Penn African Studies Workshop (October 17, 1997). http://www.africa.upenn.edu/Workshop/sara.html (20 August 2013).

Bolt, Maxim. "Waged Entrepreneurs, Policed Informality: Work, the Regulation of Space and the Economy of the Zimbabwean–South African Border." *Africa* 82, 1 (2012): 111–130.

Brown, Spencer H. "A tool of empire: The British medical establishment in Lagos, 1861–1905." *International Journal of African Historical Studies* 37, 2 (2004): 309–344.

Büscher, Karen and Gillian Mathys. "Navigating the Urban 'In-Between Space': Local Livelihood and Identity Strategies in Exploiting the Goma/Gisenyi Border." In *Violence on the Margins: States, Conflict, and Borderlands*, edited by Benedikt Korff and Timothy Raemaekers. 119–142. New York: Palgrave Macmillan, 2013.

Comaroff, Jean and John Comaroff. *Of revelation and revolution: Christianity, colonialism, and consciousness in South Africa*. Chicago: University of Chicago Press, 1991.

———. *Of revelation and revolution, Volume Two: The dialectics of modernity on a South African frontier*. Chicago: University of Chicago Press, 1997.

Cunningham, H. and J. Heyman. "Introduction: Mobilities and Enclosures at Borders." *Identities* 11, 2 (2004): 289–302.

Das, V. and D. Poole. "State and its Margins: Comparative ethnographies." In *Anthropology in the Margins of the State*, edited by V. Das and D. Poole. 3–33. New Delhi: Oxford University Press, 2004.

Digby, Anne, Waltraud Ernst, and Projit B. Mukharji, ed. *Crossing Colonial Historiographies: Histories of Colonial and Indigenous Medicines in Transnational Perspective*. Cambridge: Cambridge Scholars Publishing, 2010.

Digby, Anne and Helen Sweet. "Nurses as Cultural Brokers in Twentieth-Century South Africa." In *Plural Medicine, Tradition and Modernity, 1800–2000*, edited by Waltraud Ernst. 113–129. London: Routledge, 2002.

Doyal, L. *The Political Economy of Health*. London: Pluto Press, 1979.

Dube, Francis. "Medicine without Borders: The American Board of Commissioners for Foreign Missions in central Mozambique and eastern Zimbabwe, 1893–1920s," *OFO: Journal of Transatlantic Studies* 4, 2 (2014): 21–38.

———. "'In the Border Regions of the Territory of Rhodesia, There Is the Greatest Scourge…': The Border and East Coast Fever Control in Central Mozambique and Eastern Zimbabwe, 1901–1942," *Journal of Southern African Studies* 41, 2 (2015): 219–235.

Ernst, Waltraud, ed. *Plural Medicine, Tradition and Modernity, 1800–2000*. London: Routledge, 2002.

Farley, John. *Bilharzia: A History of Imperial Tropical Medicine*. Cambridge: Cambridge University Press, 1991.

Farmer, Paul. *Infections and Inequalities: The Modern Plagues*. Berkeley, University of California Press, 1999.

Feierman, Steven and John M. Janzen. Introduction to *The Social Basis of Health and Healing in Africa*. Berkeley: University of California Press, 1992.

Feierman, Steven. *Peasant Intellectuals: Anthropology and History in Tanzania*. Madison: University of Madison Press, 1990.

———. "Colonizers, Scholars and the Creation of Invisible Histories." In *Beyond the Cultural Turn: New Directions in the Study of Society and Culture*, edited by Victoria E. Bonnell and Lynn Hunt. 182–216. Berkeley: University of California Press, 1999.

———. "On Socially Composed Knowledge: Reconstructing a Shambaa Royal Ritual." In *In Search of a Nation: Histories of Authority and Dissidence in Tanzania*, edited by James L. Giblin and Gregory H. Maddox. 14–32. Athens: Ohio University Press, 2005.

Dissidence in Tanzania. "Struggles for Control: The Social Roots of Health and Healing in Modern Africa." *African Studies Review* 28 (1995): 73–147.

Feyissa, Dereje and Markus Virgil Hoehne. "State Borders and Borderlands as Resources." In *Borders and Borderlands as Resources in the Horn of Africa*, edited by Dereje Feyissa and Markus Virgil Hoehne. 1–7. Suffolk: James Currey, 2010.

Flint, Karen. *Healing Traditions: African Medicine, Cultural Exchange, and Competition in South Africa, 1820–1948*. Athens: Ohio University Press, 2008.

Ford, John. *The Role of the Trypanosomiases in African Ecology: A Study of the Tsetse Fly Problem*. Oxford: Clarendon Press, 1971.

Gelfand, Michael. *Proud Record in Health Services in Rhodesia and Nyasaland*. Salisbury, Southern Rhodesia, 1959.

———. *A Service to the Sick: A History of the Health Services for Africans in Southern Rhodesia, 1890–1953.* Gwelo: Mambo Press, 1976.

Gros, Jean-Germain. *Healthcare Policy in Africa: Institutions and Politics from Colonialism to the Present.* Lanham: Rowman & Littlefield, 2016.

Harries, Patrick. *Work, Culture, and Identity: Migrant Laborers in Mozambique and South Africa, c. 1860–1910.* Portsmouth, Heinemann, 1994.

Harrison, Mark. *Public Health in British India: Anglo-Indian Preventive Medicine, 1859–1914.* Cambridge: Cambridge University Press, 1994.

Hokkanen, Markku. *Medicine, Mobility and the Empire: Nyasaland Networks, 1859–1960.* Manchester: Manchester University Press, 2017.

Hughes, David M. *From Enslavement to Environmentalism: Politics on a Southern African Frontier.* Seattle: University of Washington Press in association with Weaver Press, Harare, 2006.

Janzen, John M. *The Quest for Therapy: Medical Pluralism in Lower Zaire.* Berkeley: University of California Press, 1978.

Johnson, Ryan and Amna Khalid. "Introduction." In *Public Health in the British Empire: Intermediaries, Subordinates, and the Practice of Public Health, 1850–1960*, edited by Ryan Johnson and Amna Khalid. 1–31. Routledge: New York, 2012.

Joseph, Yakubu and Rainer Rothfuss. "Symbolic Bordering and the Securitization of Identity Markers in Nigeria's Ethno-Religiously Segregated City of Jos." In *Placing the Border in Everyday Life*, edited by Reece Jones and Corey Johnson. 167–184. Surrey: Ashgate, 2014.

Korff, Benedikt and Timothy Raeymaekers. "Introductions: Border, Frontier and the Geography of Rule at the Margins of the State." In *Violence on the Margins: States, Conflict, and Borderlands*, edited by Benedikt Korff and Timothy Raemaekers. 3–27. New York: Palgrave Macmillan, 2013.

Lachenal, Guillaume. "Experimental Hubris and Medical Powerlessness: Notes from a Colonial Utopia, Cameroon, 1939–1949." In *Rethinking Biomedicine and Governance in Africa: Contributions from Anthropology*, edited by Paul Wenzel Geissler, Richard Rottenburg, and Julia Zenker. 119–140. Bielefeld: Verlag, 2012.

———. *The Lomidine Files: The Untold Story of a Medical Disaster in Colonial Africa.* Baltimore: Johns Hopkins University Press, 2017.

Last, Murray. "Understanding Health." In *Culture and Global Change*, edited by Tim Allen and Tracy Skelton. 72–86. London: Routledge, 1999.

Livingston, Julie. *Debility and the Moral Imagination in Botswana.* Bloomington: Indiana University Press, 2005.

Luedke, Tracy J. and Harry G. West. "Healing Divides: Therapeutic Border Work in Southeast Africa." In *Borders and Healers: Brokering Therapeutic Resources in Southeast Africa*, edited by Tracy J. Luedke and Harry G. West. 1–20. Bloomington, IN: Indiana University Press, 2006.

Lyons, Maryinez. "Public Health in Colonial Africa: The Belgian Congo." In *The History of Public Health and the Modern State*, edited by Dorothy Porter. 356–381. Amsterdam: Rodopi, 1994.

MacLeod, Roy. Preface to *Disease, Medicine, Empire: Perspectives on Western Medicine and the Experience of European Expansion*. New York: Routledge, 1988.

Marsland, Rebecca "Who Are the 'Public' in Public Health?: Debating Crowds, Populations, and Publics in Tanzania." In *Making and Unmaking of Public Health in Africa: Ethnographic and Historical Perspectives*, edited by Ruth J. Prince and Rebecca Marsland. 75–95. Athens: Ohio University Press, 2014.

McGovern, Mike. "Bushmeat and the Politics of Disgust." *Fieldsights – Hot Spots, Cultural Anthropology Online*. (October 07, 2014). http://www.culanth.org/fieldsights/588-bushmeat-and-the-politics-of-disgust (24 December 2014).

Menzies, R., I. Rocher, and B. Vissandjee. "Factors Associated with compliance in Treatment of Tuberculosis." *Tuberculosis and Lung Disease* 74 (1993): 32–37.

Merson, Michael H.. et al. *International Public Health: Diseases, Programs, Systems, and Policies*. Gaithersburg: Aspen Publishers, 2001.

Mohr, Adam. "Missionary Medicine and Akan Therapeutics: Illness, Health and Healing in Southern Ghana's Basel Mission, 1828–1918." *Journal of Religion in Africa* 39 (2009): 429–461.

Moran, Mary and Hoffman, Daniel. "Ebola in Perspective." *Fieldsights – Hot Spots, Cultural Anthropology Online*. (October 07, 2014) http://www.culanth.org/fieldsights/585-ebola-in-perspective (24 December 2014).

Ndege, George O. *Health, State, and Society in Kenya*. Rochester: University of Rochester Press, 2001.

Neill, Deborah. *Networks in Tropical Medicine: Internationalism, Colonialism, and the Rise of a Medical Specialty, 1890–1930*. Palo Alto: Stanford University Press, 2012.

Orwell, George. "How the Poor Die." (November, 1946) http://orwell.ru/library/articles/Poor_Die/english/e_pdie (8 August 2014).

Packard, Randall M. "Visions of Postwar Health and Development and Their Impact on Public Health Interventions in the Developing World." In *Internal Development and the Social Sciences: Essays on the History and Politics of Knowledge*, edited by Fredrick Cooper and Randall Packard. 93–115. Berkeley: University of California Press, 1997.

Patton, Adell Jr. *Physicians, Colonial Racism, and Diaspora in West Africa*. Gainesville: University of Florida, 1996.

Porter, Roy. *The Greatest Benefit to Mankind: A Medical History of Humanity*. New York: W. W. Norton & Company, 1997.

Prince, Ruth J. "Introduction: Situating Health and the Public in Africa." In *Making and Unmaking of Public Health in Africa: Ethnographic and Historical Perspectives*, edited by Ruth J. Prince and Rebecca Marsland. 1–51. Athens: Ohio University Press, 2014.

Renne, Elisha P. "Parallel Dilemmas: Polio Transmission and Political Violence in Northern Nigeria." *Africa* 84, 3 (2014): 466–486.

———. *The Politics of Polio in Northern Nigeria*. Bloomington: Indiana University Press, 2010.

Richards, Paul and Alfred Mokuwa. "Village Funerals and the Spread of Ebola Virus Disease." *Fieldsights – Hot Spots, Cultural Anthropology Online*. (October 07, 2014). http://www.culanth.org/fieldsights/590-village-funerals-and-the-spread-of-ebola-virus-disease (24 December 2014).

Roque, Ana Cristina. "A History of Mozambique's Southern Border: The Archives of the Portuguese Commission of Cartography." In *Borderlands and Frontiers in Africa*, edited by Steven Van Wolputte. 23–54. Berlin: LIT VERLAG Dr. W. Hopf, 2013.

Rose, Hunt, Nancy. *A Colonial Lexicon: Of Birth Ritual, Medicalization, and Mobility in the Congo*. Durham: Duke University Press, 1999.

Rutherford, Blair. "The Politics of Boundaries: The Shifting Terrain of Belonging for Zimbabweans in a South African Border Zone." *African Diaspora: Transnational Journal of Culture, Economy & Society* 4, 2 (2011): 207–229.

Sadowsky, Jonathan. *Imperial Bedlam: Institutions of Madness and Colonialism in Southwest Nigeria*. Berkeley: University of California Press, 1999.

———. "The long Shadow of Colonialism: Why We Study Medicine in Africa." In *Medicine and Healing in Africa: Multidisciplinary Perspectives*, edited by Paula Viterbo and Kalala Ngalamulume. 210–217. East Lansing: Michigan State University Press, 2010.

Shamir, Ronen. "Without Borders? Notes on Globalization as a Mobility Regime." *Sociological Theory* 23, 2 (2005): 197–217.

Shapiro, Martin. "Medicine in the Service of Colonialism: Medical Care in Portuguese Africa, 1885–1974." Ph.D. Thesis, University of California, Los Angeles, 1983.

Scott, James. *Weapons of the Weak: Everyday Forms of Peasant Resistance*. Yale University Press: New Haven, CT, 1985.

Tsing, Ana L. "From the Margins." *Cultural Anthropology* 9, 3 (1994): 279–297.

van Schendel, W. "Spaces of Engagement: How Borderlands, Illegal Flows and Territorial States Interlock." In *Illicit Flows and Criminal Things: States, Borders, and the Other Side of Globalization*, edited by I. Abraham and W. van Schendel. 38–68. Bloomington IN, Indiana University Press, 2005.

Vaughan, Megan. *Curing Their Ills: Colonial Power and African Illness*. Stanford: Stanford University Press, 1993.

———. "Healing and Curing Issues in the Social History and Anthropology of Medicine in Africa." *Social History of Medicine* 7, 2 (1994): 283–295.

Waite, Gloria. "Public Health in Pre-colonial East-Central Africa." In *The Social Basis of Health and Healing in Africa*, edited Steven Feierman and John M. Janzen. 212–231. Berkeley: University of California Press, 1992.

Webb, James L. A. Jr. "The First Large-Scale Use of Synthetic Insecticide for Malaria Control in Tropical Africa: Lessons from Liberia, 1945–62." In *Global Health in Africa: Historical Perspectives on Disease*, edited by James L. A. Webb, Jr. and Tamara Giles-Vernick. 42–69. Athens: Ohio University Press, 2013.

White, Luise. *Speaking with Vampires: Rumor and History in Colonial Africa*. Berkeley: University of California Press, 2000.

Worboys, Michael. "The Emergence of Tropical Medicine." *Perspectives on the Emergence of Scientific Disciplines*, edited by Gerard Lemaine, Roy Macleod, and Michael Mulkay. 75–98, The Hague: Mouton, 1976.

———. "The Discovery of Colonial Malnutrition between the Wars." *Imperial Medicine and Indigenous Societies*, edited by David Arnold. 208–223. Manchester: Manchester University Press, 1988.

PART I

Life and Health Before the Border

CHAPTER 2

The Trans-border Landscape: Regional Mobility and Health Before the Border

An examination of the social, political, and economic history of the agrarian societies of the Shona people and patterns of mobility shows why villagers would have traveled. Villagers traveled for a number of reasons, including traveling to visit family and kin, to trade, to hunt, and for health reasons, among other reasons. In addition, the organization of precolonial "public health" largely overlapped with environmental differences, with people in semi-arid areas concerned about rainfall, harvest, food security, and health, for example. Health-wise, traveling was a way of gaining or maintaining health through visiting healers, moving to different environments, visiting spirit mediums and shrines, as well as through healers traveling to treat patients or to find medicines. Therefore, free circulation of people and interconnections across the region for purposes of trade, exchanging complementary products, keeping kinship connections alive, hunting, gathering medicines, and many other reasons were vital.

The area under focus in Zimbabwe stretches from Pungwe (Pungué) River in the north, then south to where the Save (Sabi) River crosses into Mozambique (see Fig. 2.1). Its western edge is demarcated by the Odzi and Save Rivers in Zimbabwe and it encloses the Mutare (Umtali), Chimanimani (North Melsetter), and Chipinge (Melsetter/Chipinga/South Melsetter) districts. In Mozambique it roughly encompasses the western portions of Manica (Macequece/Masekesa/Massi-Kessi, also known as (Vila de) Manhiça), Sussundenga, and Mossurize (Musirizwi/Umselezwe/Umsilizi/Mossurise) districts. This border region generally

F. Dube, *Public Health at the Border of Zimbabwe and Mozambique, 1890–1940*, African Histories and Modernities,
https://doi.org/10.1007/978-3-030-47535-2_2

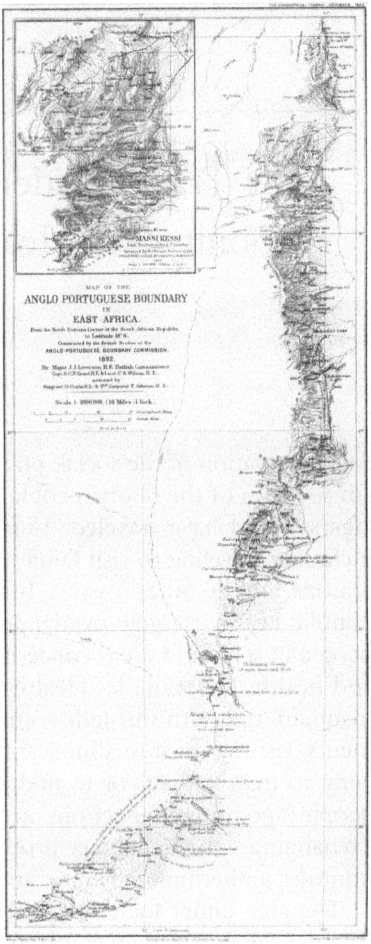

Fig. 2.1 Map of the Zimbabwe-Mozambique border region. (Reproduced with permission from *The Geographical Journal* 2, 6 (1893))

falls into areas inhabited by the eastern Shona people, with the Manyika in the north and the Ndau in the south.[1] The major urban centers are Mutare, Penhalonga (a gold mining town), Chipinge, and Chimanimani in Zimbabwe. The major towns on the Mozambican side are Manica, Espungabera in Mossurize district, and Sussundenga.

The Zimbabwe-Mozambique border region's physical attributes had a profound effect on settlement patterns, farming, livestock-keeping, disease, and patterns of mobility. It is an area of high elevation, particularly on the Zimbabwean side, which meant that this Zimbabwean side was less susceptible to tsetse fly and trypanosomiasis. Consequently, villagers practiced a form of transhumance, keeping their livestock on the highlands of Zimbabwe during the rainy season and moving the animals to the lowlands of Mozambique during the dry season when pastures were scarce on the highlands and when the threat of trypanosomiasis in the lowland decreased due to low temperatures. In fact, the Zimbabwe-Mozambique international border follows the crest of the Vumba range of mountains to the north and the Chimanimani range of mountains to the south. Known as the Eastern Highlands in Zimbabwe, this region's natural fertility, land, and water-based routes have profoundly influenced its history.[2]

The fertile soils, mineral resources, vegetation, and livestock-rearing potential attracted both African and, later, European settlements. Land in Zimbabwe has been classified into "natural farming regions" I–V, with region I being the most productive agricultural land with high rainfall and V being an arid environment, with little agricultural potential. The Zimbabwean side of the border region has some of the best farmlands ranging from "natural farming regions" I–II. These are healthy upland plateaus around Chimanimani and Chipinge at around 3937–7874 feet (1200–2400 meters) above sea level. The region has deep, reddish brown sandy loam soils that cover the Eastern Highlands to as far north as Nyanga (Inyanga). These soils have good moisture retention capacity, a characteristic essential for ensuring adequate moisture for growth of plants. The highland peoples were therefore able to produce surplus food, which was traded with the less fortunate peoples of the lowlands. According to Robin

[1] For an extended discussion of Ndau history over the *longue durée*, see Elizabeth MacGonagle, *Crafting Identity in Zimbabwe and Mozambique* (Rochester: University of Rochester Press, 2007).

[2] John Keith Rennie, "Christianity, Colonialism and the Origins of Nationalism among the Ndau of Southern Rhodesia, 1890–1935," PhD Thesis, Department of History, Northwestern University, 1973, 37.

Palmer, there was much local trade in the region, "for example in the Melsetter area between the people of the drought-stricken Sabi Valley, who in bad years exchanged salt, dried fish, palm wine, mats, baskets, and cloth for grain and tobacco from the people of the more favoured uplands."[3] Similarly, Jocelyn Alexander notes that the economy of Chimanimani was more dependent on local trade between the larger villages of the mountains and the scattered lowland settlements, driven by *shangwa* (drought and disaster), than on long-distance trade in cattle and ivory.[4]

Besides the quality of the soils, other factors crucial for plant growth and animal domestication are rainfall and temperature. The highlands of the border region receive annual rainfall of between 45 and 55 inches, which is higher than in any other region in Zimbabwe and reliable, thanks to light winter rains. The temperatures in the highlands are also comfortable and conducive to crop production all year round, with the mean daily temperature averaging between 55 and 70 °F (12.77 and 21.11 °C).

Apart from climatic factors, rivers associated with the border region also played a role in the social and economic history of the Shona peoples. The presence of water encouraged the growth of thickets of vegetation, which in some areas harbored tsetse flies. Rivers also impacted travel, fishing, and farming. The major rivers of the region are the Save, Odzi, Pungwe, Budzi (Busi/Búzi), Musirizwi, Rusitu (Lucite), Harondi (Chibira/Harom), Mussapa, and Rebvuwe (Revuè). The Pungwe rises in the Nyanga Mountains, whose peaks rise to over 8500 feet (2590.8 meters) and flows in a southeasterly direction to the Indian Ocean. It is largely "a rapid mountain river" until it enters a flat area toward the Indian Ocean.[5] The Budzi originates in the table-land north of Chief Mapungwana's (Mapungane) area and flows in a southeasterly direction to its confluence with the Musirizwi. The Rebvuwe also rises in the mountains and follows an easterly direction to the Indian Ocean.

Another river of importance, the Mussapa, originates in an area north of the Chimanimani Mountains and flows in a southeasterly direction to its confluence with the Rusitu. The Rusitu, flowing in a deep valley with

[3] Robin Palmer, *Land and Racial Domination in Rhodesia* (Berkeley: University of California Press, 1977), 14.

[4] Jocelyn Alexander, *The Unsettled Land: State-Making and the Politics of Land in Zimbabwe* (Athens: Ohio University Press, 2006), 19.

[5] J. J. Leverson, "Geographical Results of the Anglo-Portuguese Delimitation Commission," *The Geographical Journal* 2, 6 (1893): 506.

mountains on its northern bank, follows an easterly direction toward the Indian Ocean. J. J. Leverson of the 1892 Anglo-Portuguese Delimitation Commission described the right bank of the Rusitu as less mountainous, being covered with "luxuriant tropical vegetation, in which clearances had been made here and there for the cultivation of mealies [corn] and other kinds of grain."[6] The other important rivers are the Chibira and the Musirizwi. While Leverson described the Chibira River as "a fierce mountain torrent," flowing southward along the foot of the craggy and precipitous western ridge of the Chimanimani Range, the Musirizwi ran through a mountain gorge which widened considerably in some places. This gave room for African villages and fields of corn (maize) as well as "Kaffir corn" (a Southern African variety of sorghum), along the river banks.[7]

Although there are no classifications of farming regions on the Mozambican side of the border, the lands adjacent to Zimbabwe's Eastern Highlands are also of high elevation. In the districts of Sussundenga and Mossurize, between the Budzi and Rusitu Rivers, for instance, the Chimanimani Mountains have a peak of over 7000 feet (2133.6 meters) and there are also massive peaks on the Matibi highlands. The most prominent feature is the straight, high narrow Sitatonga Ridge that "pointing to the magnetic north, cuts at right angles to the two rivers [Budzi and Rusitu] and effectively shuts off the lowland plains east of it from the foothill and valley country to its west."[8] In general, the elevation ranges from well over 4000 feet (1219.2 meters) on Mount Umtareni and the Sitatonga crests, and 3700 feet (1127.7 meters) at Espungabera, to 2000 and 1000 feet (609.6 and 304.8 meters) and less in the lower valleys between the Sitatongas and the Zimbabwean border. East of the Sitatongas, the general elevation falls to around 500–600 feet (152.4–182.8 meters) above sea level.

The region's physical and climatic characteristics influenced agricultural patterns. In the northern parts of the border region, in what was the Manyika Kingdom, precolonial villagers grew a variety of crops two or three times a year. The relief of the area from the coast to Manica caused the rainy season and mists to last for a long time.[9] This complicated con-

[6] Ibid., 509.

[7] Ibid., 510.

[8] C. F. M. Swynnerton, "Examination of the tsetse problem in North Mossurise, Portuguese East Africa," *Bulletin of Entomological Research* 11, no. 4 (1921): 318.

[9] H. H. K. Bhila, *Trade and Politics in a Shona Kingdom: the Manyika and their African and Portuguese Neighbours, 1575–1902* (Essex: Longman, 1982), 6.

trol of a number of livestock diseases, particularly East Coast Fever during the colonial period because such mists lingering for weeks made it difficult to hunt down and dip cattle to kill off disease-carrying ticks. From the coast, the terrain over 186 miles (300 km) gradually rises until it reaches an altitude of 2297 feet (700.1 meters) and then suddenly rises to elevations varying between 4921 and 6562 feet (1499.9 and 2000 meters) above sea level. Relief rainfall is common in this region as the humid winds from the Indian Ocean condense rapidly to deliver torrential rains. The humid areas close to the coast harbored trypanosomiasis vectors, tsetse flies, making cattle-keeping difficult. Leverson claimed that the whole area from the Pungwe River to Shimoya's (Chimoio, east of Manica, also known as Vila Pery or Vila Chimoro) was tsetse fly infested.[10]

The highland rivers valleys are fertile and capable of supporting dense populations, but fertility decreases as one moves south toward the Save River valley, an area of low and uncertain rainfall with poor drainage and saline soils. This is because south of the Musirizwi River, the land becomes less mountainous, drier, and sandy, forming "a gently undulating district covered with grass and stunted trees."[11] The same situation applies to the Zimbabwean side of the border as one moves from the Eastern Highlands to the west toward the Save River. To the west of the fertile highlands, in a broad north-south strip parallel to the Save River, the natural farming region classification ranges between III and V. The soils become less and less fertile with low and unreliable rainfall, often punctuated by periodic droughts. Crop failures were common, contributing to regular travel to the highlands to trade for food. The valley floor forms a broad flat sandy plain with elevations of between 1000 and 2000 feet. Here the alluvial soils are fertile but rainfall is generally below 24 inches per year and is extremely unreliable and temperatures can rise well to over 100 °F. (37.77 °C) in summer.

The nature of the land and climate influenced vegetation patterns in the region, which in turn affected disease ecology. Around Mutare and Mozambique's Manica district, forests, which influence the distribution of tsetse flies, were of a thin and open character, with a few patches of dense tropical forest. The trees were mostly deciduous with the main product of the forest being rubber from the natural vines, *Landolphia*, which grew

[10] Leverson, "Geographical Results of the Anglo-Portuguese Delimitation Commission," 517.

[11] Ibid., 510.

over wide areas.[12] The mountains were mostly grass covered. In general, proceeding from the border to the east in Mozambique, the land drops from a heavily forested plateau of about 3000 feet (914.4 meters) above sea level to a broad low coastal plain. Rainfall in the highlands ranges from 35 to 70 inches per annum, providing adequate moisture for plant growth.

While surveying the border region in 1892, Leverson observed that forests were common, particularly along the mountain slopes exposed to high rainfall, and were covered by the common *brachystegia* (*Msasa* trees), whereas the lowlands were characterized by Mopane bush. "Mount Venga, just to the north of Massi-Kessi, and a few other peaks are covered with trees to their summits," he noted, "but the greater portion of the very high ground is grass land, while the valleys, except that of the Revuè, and the plains are nearly everywhere covered with forest."[13] He also observed that the slopes of the mountains enclosing the Rusitu River gorge were for the most part covered with thick forest, while the plains and valleys of the area north of the Save were covered with mopane (acacia) forest.

The Zimbabwe-Mozambique border region had a variety of wild animals including elephants, antelope, wild pig, buffalo, carnivores, and smaller animals, which influenced hunting patterns and the epidemiology of vector-borne disease, including trypanosomiasis (sleeping sickness). It had large herds of elephants to the extent that the Mutema people, whose capital was traditionally at Ngaone (about 30 miles (48.28 kilometers at an elevation of 4960.63 feet or 1512 meters) from the border) in the Eastern Highlands, are remembered as the people who "ruled with ivory."[14] Leverson observed that from Manica in the north to the Save in the south, much of the region's game existed between the Chimanimani Pass and the Musirizwi Rivers.[15] This included eland, buffalo, hartebeest, wildebeest, bushbuck, reedbuck, quagga, sable antelope, blue buck, red antelope, and wild boar. These similarities and variations in physical features, vegetation, and wildlife influenced the prevalence and control of diseases, such as trypanosomiasis discussed in Chap. 5.

The region was also rich in mineral deposits including gold in the north, particularly around the Penhalonga area, north of Mutare in

[12] Bhila, *Trade and Politics in a Shona Kingdom*, 7.

[13] Leverson, "Geographical Results of the Anglo-Portuguese Delimitation Commission," 513.

[14] Bhila, *Trade and Politics in a Shona Kingdom*, 2.

[15] Leverson, "Geographical Results of the Anglo-Portuguese Delimitation Commission," 518.

Zimbabwe, and in parts of Manica district in Mozambique. H. H. K. Bhila has noted that of the four major gold producing regions, the Rebvuwe, Mutari, Nyamukwarara, and Munene Rivers and their tributaries, the richest gold deposits were those of the Rebvuwe River and its tributaries.[16] Apart from these areas, alluvial gold was found in the Penhalonga valley.[17] This mining potential influenced colonization of the region in the 1890s, with both the Portuguese and British vying for the region's mineral wealth. The region also possessed coal, iron, and copper deposits. Mining was therefore common in the northern parts of the area, in Manica district of Mozambique and in areas around Mutare in Zimbabwe.

Communication was by way of the Pungwe River, navigable for about a hundred miles, and also by the Save River, navigable from the Indian Ocean up to the Zimbabwean border. In addition, there were numerous land routes, some of which followed river valleys from Zimbabwe all the way to the coast in the east. Hence the colonial border did not enclose natural communication areas, but divided them and bisected the routes to the coast.[18]

The Eastern Shona in Precolonial Times

The ancestors of the Shona people settled on the Zimbabwean plateau in the fifth century CE and practiced mining, agriculture, and livestock production. The following centuries witnessed flourishing trade in gold and ivory with Arab trading posts on the East African coast contributing to considerable expansion of Shona culture. The basic social structure of African society in the border region comprised extended families and lineage groups clustered in villages. The sizes of these villages varied according to the physical conditions of the area. The most densely populated areas were Zinyumbu, the Musirizwi-Budzi basin, and Mafuse (Mafusi) as these were rich agricultural areas with plenty of rainfall.[19] Leverson noted the variations in population density of the region in 1892. "Journeying south from Massi-Kessi it [population] is very sparse as far as the Chimanimani mountains," he observed, "very little is obtainable in the way of food supplies. The Natives have no cattle, and appear to live in the

[16] Bhila, *Trade and Politics in a Shona Kingdom*, 41.
[17] Bhila, *Trade and Politics in a Shona Kingdom*, 42.
[18] Rennie, "Christianity, Colonialism and the Origins of Nationalism," 41.
[19] Bhila, *Trade and Politics in a Shona Kingdom*, 2.

dread of a raid by Gungunyane [ruler of the Gaza state based in Mozambique]."[20] Leverson observed, however, that there was more cultivation and probably more people in the Mussapa River valley.

Another densely populated area was the land between the Rusitu and Musirizwi Rivers in the south. Leverson claimed that this was the most densely populated and prosperous part of the border region, where villages were bigger, with much better built houses, more cultivation, and large numbers of fowls reared than anywhere else.[21] All this contributed to an air of well-being and comfort. Another indication of the high population density was that in the more fertile highlands, the population was concentrated in large villages of up to 40 huts such that the more scattered populations to the south sometimes referred to the highlanders as *vaguta* (town dwellers).[22] However, south of the Musirizwi River the area became less fertile and the population diminished again.

The precolonial economy of the border region included crop and livestock production. When J. J. Leverson visited the region in 1892, he noted that Africans cultivated several crops including bananas, the castor-oil plant, chili peppers, tomatoes, sweet potatoes, groundnuts (peanuts), mealies (maize/corn), "Kaffir corn," and various kinds of African grain such as red oofoo, tobacco, and non-poisonous manioc (cassava).[23]

Apart from agriculture, livestock-keeping was also a major economic activity. In fact, Malyn Newitt noted, for their wealth and status, the rulers of the plateau states relied far more on cattle than on foreign trade.[24] Leverson claimed in 1892 that Chief Mapungwana of the southern part of the border region had some cattle which thrived on the high plateau, where his main *kraal* (village) was situated. In the northern portion of the region, he reported seeing cattle on the high ground in the catchment areas of the Odzi and Mutare streams, where there were no tsetse flies, the vectors responsible for spreading trypanosomiasis. Leverson also noted the absence of tsetse in the Rebvuwe and Menini River valleys into which

[20] Leverson, "Geographical Results of the Anglo-Portuguese Delimitation Commission," 515.

[21] Ibid., 515–516.

[22] Rennie, "Christianity, Colonialism and the Origins of Nationalism," 54.

[23] Leverson, "Geographical Results of the Anglo-Portuguese Delimitation Commission," 515. "Oofoo" is a kind of millet, see Alice Blanke Balfour, *Twelve hundred miles in a wagon* (London: Edward Arnold, 1895), 143.

[24] Malyn Newitt, *A History of Mozambique* (Bloomington: Indiana University Press, 1995), 36.

Europeans had recently imported cattle.[25] However, he reported encounters with the tsetse fly in the Save River area, making it challenging to keep cattle in this area.

The analysis of marriage practices in the border region also confirms cattle-raising as a major economic activity. In the fertile and densely populated areas suitable for cattle, such as the highlands, cattle were central in marriage transactions. However, in the drier or more mountainous areas less suitable for cattle, such as the Chimanimani chieftaincies of Hodi, Nyamazha, Gariyadza, and Saungweme, a man did not need cattle to marry. In these chieftaincies a man could obtain a wife by becoming a *mugariri* (son-in-law with labor obligations to the woman's father).[26] This practice was also more common among the Danda (Sedanda) in the less fertile area between the Save and Budzi Rivers in Mozambique than among the Chisanga (Quissanga/Sanga) of the highlands in Chipinge, Zimbabwe.

As a result of this environmental diversity, movements to procure various resources were common in the precolonial period. As Malyn Newitt notes, in the sixteenth century as in the twentieth century African societies of the border region were susceptible to drought and famine, with gold producers using cloth and beads obtained from coastal traders to buy grain or cattle from neighbors with surpluses.[27] A 1537 Portuguese document, for instance, suggests that the Manyika used imported trade goods to buy food from the Quiteve and Baroe because the Manyika preferred trade to agriculture.[28]

Apart from these movements to find food, there were many other reasons contributing to high rates of mobility in the region. Villagers also traveled to visit family members and relatives, to hunt, for both commercial and subsistence purposes, for health reasons, and transhumance. Healers traveled to find medicines available only in certain micro-environments and they also traveled to visit patients. Villagers traveled to healers, which they still do to this day. Others traveled to visit spirit mediums to find answers to a variety of questions, including ill health. Hence, there were a number of factors that contributed to mobility in the region.

[25] Leverson, "Geographical Results of the Anglo-Portuguese Delimitation Commission," 516.

[26] Rennie, "Christianity, Colonialism and the Origins of Nationalism," 54.

[27] Newitt, *A History of Mozambique*, 51.

[28] Ibid.

The villages sometimes coalesced into empires and chiefdoms. On the Zimbabwean plateau several empires emerged including Great Zimbabwe (1200–1450), the Mwenemutapa (Mutapa) Empire (c. 1450–1629), both of which extended hegemony to most parts of present-day central Mozambique, and later the Rozvi Empire of Changamire Dombo in the seventeenth century. At the zenith of its power, the Mwenemutapa Empire controlled vast areas, from the plateau to the east coast, through vassal states like Danda, Chisanga, Quiteve, Manica (Manyika), Báruè (Barwe), and many others.[29] Thus when the Portuguese explorer Vasco da Gama landed on the East African coast in 1498, Mozambique was the point of contact between two of the most powerful and highly developed civilizations in Africa—the trade-oriented Swahili (Muslim) culture of the east coast and the culture of Zimbabwe, which specialized in metal processing. The coming of the Portuguese into the region contributed to the decline of the flourishing Indian Ocean trade and African cultures experienced a gradual transformation as they interacted with the Portuguese who sought to control the sources of gold in the region. Hence, beginning in the last quarter of the sixteenth century to the late seventeenth century, "there was an extensive and interlocking network of trade between the [Portuguese] feiras in Makaranga, Butwa and Manyika."[30] The Portuguese went on to establish their presence in Mozambique through the institution of *prazos* in Tete and Sena, for instance, and also by establishing garrisons at Inhambane, Sofala, Villa de Manica, Sena, and Tete.[31] The Portuguese also attempted to control gold trade. This knowledge of the presence of gold in the region later provided an incentive for the formal colonization of the area.

The Shona people of the Zimbabwe-Mozambique border region, including the Manyika in the north and the Ndau in the south, probably formed part of the Mbire state in the eighteenth century. The Mbire was a successor state to the Mwenemutapa Empire. The Manyika Kingdom in

[29] C. Serra, *História de Moçambique*, volume 1, (Maputo: Livraria Universitária, 2000), 35.

[30] Bhila, *Trade and Politics in a Shona Kingdom*, 81.

[31] *Prazos* were large estates leased to Portuguese colonial settlers and traders. They operated in a semi-feudal fashion and were common in the Zambezi River valley, north of the border region. For more on the activities of the Portuguese before formal colonial rule, see M. D. D. Newitt, *Portuguese Settlement on the Zambesi: Exploration, Land Tenure, and Colonial Rule in East Africa* (New York: African Publishing Company, 1973) and Allen Isaacman, *Mozambique: The Africanization of a European Institution; the Zambesi Prazos, 1750–1902* (Madison: University of Wisconsin Press, 1972).

the northern mountainous region, though small, was of great antiquity.[32] First ruled by the Chikanga dynasty, this kingdom was then ruled by the Mutasa dynasty in the early nineteenth century before the British and the Portuguese partitioned the entire area between themselves in 1891.[33]

In the southern part of the border region, among the Ndau, a number of polities emerged in the seventeenth century. These included the Dziva chieftaincies of Musikavanhu, Mapungwana, Makuyana, Sahodi (Ngorima), Saungweme (Chikume), Mutambara, and Chirimugwenzi (Gwenzi), Mafuse, Gogoyo (Gogoi), and Chisanga, whose rulers were known by the dynastic title Mutema.[34]

By the late nineteenth century, however, these polities had effectively disintegrated, except Barwe, although some remnants remained in the chiefdoms of M'cupi in Danda, Manica in Macequece, and Moribane in Quiteve.[35] Most of the region's polities had suffered at the hands of Zwangendaba and Soshangana (Manikusi), Nguni generals who fled from Shaka in Natal during the *Mfecane*. The *Mfecane* was the dispersal of the Nguni people of Natal which began in the early nineteenth century. Soshangane and his Shangani people established the Gaza state with its capital at Bileni, on Delagoa Bay (later called Lourenço Marques and now the Mozambican capital, Maputo). However, in order to get farther away from Natal, Soshangane moved north in 1828 with his army of followers and asserted his authority north of the Save River as far as the Mussapa. He defeated Nxaba and Zwangendaba (two other Nguni generals who had preceded him) and subdued the surrounding peoples, including Portuguese garrisons at Inhambane, Sofala, Villa de Manica, Sena, and Tete. He then established his empire of Gazaland with its capital in the Musirizwi valley and was succeeded by his son, Mzila, in 1860. Mzila's reign witnessed the resurgence of Portuguese power and when Mzila died in 1885, his son and successor, Gungunyana, unsuccessfully attempted to play off the British and Portuguese against one another.[36] In 1889, Gungunyana evacuated Gazaland and moved his capital to the lower Limpopo, which was his grandfather's old capital at Bileni. However, the Portuguese found a pretext for attacking him between 1895 and 1897.

[32] Newitt, *Portuguese Settlement on the Zambesi*, 25.

[33] Ibid.

[34] Rennie, "Christianity, Colonialism and the Origins of Nationalism," 65–71.

[35] Barry Neil-Tomlinson, "The Mozambique Chartered Company, 1892 to 1910," PhD Thesis, School of Oriental and African Studies, University of London, 1987, 11.

[36] Ford, *The Role of the Trypanosomiases in African Ecology*, 334.

The Portuguese defeated Gungunyana and exiled him to the Canary Islands and effectively dismantled the Gaza Empire, eliminating the remaining obstacle to effective European occupation of the region.

It is clear, therefore, that there were complex networks of interdependence in this Zimbabwe-Mozambique border region before the imposition of the border after 1890. In an area with such a diversity of environments, travel was crucial to obtaining various kinds of resources. The imposition of the border would, however, disrupt all these networks, including healing networks and precolonial public health.

References

Alexander, Jocelyn. *The Unsettled Land: State-making and the Politics of Land in Zimbabwe, 1893–2003.* Oxford: James Currey, 2006.

Balfour, Alice Blanke. *Twelve Hundred Miles in a Wagon.* London: Edward Arnold, 1895.

Bhila, H. H. K. *Trade and Politics in a Shona Kingdom: The Manyika and Their African and Portuguese Neighbours, 1575–1902.* Essex: Longman, 1982.

Ford, John. *The Role of the Trypanosomiases in African Ecology: A Study of the Tsetse Fly Problem.* Oxford: Clarendon Press, 1971.

Isaacman, Allen. *Mozambique: The Africanization of a European Institution; the Zambesi Prazos, 1750–1902.* Madison, University of Wisconsin Press, 1972.

Leverson, J. J. "Geographical Results of the Anglo-Portuguese Delimitation Commission." *The Geographical Journal* 2, no. 6 (1893): 505–518.

MacGonagle, Elizabeth. *Crafting Identity in Zimbabwe and Mozambique.* Rochester: University of Rochester Press, 2007.

Neil-Tomlinson, Barry. "The Mozambique Chartered Company, 1892 to 1910." PhD Thesis, School of Oriental and African Studies, University of London, 1987.

Newitt, M. D. D. *Portuguese Settlement on the Zambesi: Exploration, Land Tenure, and Colonial Rule in East Africa.* New York: African Publishing Company, 1973.

Newitt, Malyn. *A History of Mozambique.* Bloomington: Indiana University Press, 1995.

Palmer, Robin. *Land and Racial Domination in Rhodesia.* Berkeley: University of California Press, 1977.

Rennie, John Keith. "Christianity, Colonialism and the Origins of Nationalism Among the Ndau of Southern Rhodesia, 1890–1935." PhD Thesis, Department of History, Northwestern University, 1973.

Serra, C. *História de Moçambique*, volume 1. Maputo: Livraria Universitária, 2000.

Swynnerton, C. F. M. "Examination of the Tsetse Problem in North Mossurise, Portuguese East Africa." *Bulletin of Entomological Research* 11, no. 4 (1921): 315–385.

PART II

Life and Health with the Border

CHAPTER 3

The Imposition of the Border and the Creation of a Public Health Problem

The Zimbabwe-Mozambique border runs along a crest of mountains, which Europeans took to be communication barriers. However, there were passes and drainage systems that facilitated communication and cultural uniformity. In this respect, therefore, the border was drawn arbitrarily because it was not reflective of long-term historical realities in the region but was merely a product of the 1891 Anglo-Portuguese Treaty.[1] It is important, therefore, to examine the process of colonization, the establishment of Christian mission stations, the demarcation of the border in 1891, as well as the scale of cross-border mobility and the bureaucratic control of these movements. The focus here is on the making of the border as a public health problem. The colonial border became a public health problem in three respects. First, as shown in Chap. 2, the organization of precolonial public health largely overlapped with environmental differences, which explains the continuing need to cross the border which artificially divided environmental zones. Second, colonial public health initiatives were confined by the colonial borders in a region whose epidemiology was fundamentally defined by cross-border movements. Third, before the border, traveling was a way of gaining or maintaining health. Hence, the bureaucratic control of the border during the colonial period

[1] For an extended discussion of Mozambique-Zimbabwe relations, see Nedson Pophiwa, "The Political and Economic Relations between Mozambique and Zimbabwe, 1890s to the present: A Literature Review" (unpublished paper, University of Zimbabwe, 2005), p. 4.

F. Dube, *Public Health at the Border of Zimbabwe and Mozambique, 1890–1940*, African Histories and Modernities,
https://doi.org/10.1007/978-3-030-47535-2_3

was dangerous to the health of African villagers. The implications of the border for the control of specific diseases are dealt with in Part III. As this chapter shows, the imposition of the border and the oppressive nature of settler colonialism conspired to make life unbearable for the Shona people of this border region.

The Zimbabwe-Mozambique Border Region During the Scramble for Africa

As in the rest of Africa in the 1880s, in the Zimbabwe-Mozambique border region, there was a race among European powers to claim territory. The contest was between the British and the Portuguese. Although the Portuguese had been in East Africa since the fifteenth century, their presence in Mozambique in 1890 was confined to a few posts on the coast and up the Zambezi River, having little influence in the life of the region's African population.[2] However, the scramble changed everything. With the call at the Berlin Conference in 1885 to make good the claims made on paper by way of "effective occupation," the Portuguese and the British clashed in their attempts to occupy the region.

British efforts were championed by the British South Africa Company (hereafter BSAC) under Cecil John Rhodes, while Portuguese colonialism was led by the Mozambique Company. Whereas Britain was motivated by expansive imperialist ideology and growing financial interests of its private citizens, as well as the need to secure a port for her territories, Portugal drew its impetus "not only from hope for financial gain, but also from a nostalgic, almost manifest destiny-like belief in its 'right'—as the (European) 'discoverer' of the region—to claim the territory."[3]

The bone of contention was the border region's goldfields which the Portuguese had made famous by their writings. Indeed, Cecil John Rhodes's motive for colonizing present-day Zimbabwe was the quest for a "second Rand," vast goldfields just like Rand goldfields of the Transvaal in South Africa. The Portuguese had known about the Zimbabwe-Mozambique border region's goldfields from the time they established themselves in East Africa. However, their initial attempts to seize them

[2] Neil-Tomlinson, "The Mozambique Chartered Company, 1892 to 1910," 2.

[3] Eric Allina-Pisano, "Negotiating Colonialism: Africans, the State, and the Market in Manica District, Mozambique, 1895–c. 1935" (PhD Dissertation, Yale University, May 2002), 47–48.

before the scramble failed. They renewed their efforts to control these fields in the 1870s and 1890s. Beginning in 1878 Portugal leased huge pieces of land to trading companies which used conscripted African labor.[4] Among these was the Mozambique Company, which was conceived as a mining enterprise. Nonetheless, the Anglo-Portuguese Treaty of July 1890 effectively excluded much of the border region's mineral resources from the Mozambique Company's territory.[5]

However, both companies soon found that the much hoped for gold deposits were scattered and difficult to extract, unlike the Rand mines of the Transvaal in South Africa. The companies therefore directed some of their efforts to agriculture and cattle-rearing, with the Mozambique Company, in particular, adopting a policy of granting large sub-concessions to individuals and companies in return for a share of their profits.[6]

The American Board of Commissioners for Foreign Missions

The analysis of the impact of colonial public health and Western medicine would be incomplete without an examination of the contribution of the American Board of Commissioners for Foreign Missions (commonly known as the American Board Mission among the Shona) in the southern part of the border region. The American Board Mission was founded in 1810, and it became the first American Christian foreign mission agency.[7] It went on to establish its earliest mission stations around the world between 1812 and 1840.[8] Among its many commitments were evangelism, Bible translation, education, and medical care. However, with evangelism's priority diminishing over time, the American Board Mission morphed into the United Church Board for World Missions in 1961. Subsequent to this, the United Church Board for World Missions became

[4] Ndege, *Culture and Customs of Mozambique*, 8.

[5] Allina-Pisano, "Negotiating Colonialism," 40.

[6] See Dube, "'In the Border Regions of the territory of Rhodesia, There is the Greatest Scourge ....'"

[7] American Board of Commissioners for Foreign Missions archives, Houghton Library, Harvard College Library, http://oasis.lib.harvard.edu/oasis/deliver/~hou01467 (November 18, 2012).

[8] Charles A. Maxfield, "The Formation and Early History of the American Board of Commissioners for Foreign Missions," 2001, http://www.maxfieldbooks.com/ABCFM.html (September 14, 2013).

the Wider Church Ministries of the United Church of Christ in the year 2000. The American Board Mission founded mission stations in South Africa in the 1830s, one in what became the Transvaal and another among the Zulu.[9] Its mission in eastern Zimbabwe and central Mozambique, known as the East Central Africa Mission, was an extension of the Zulu mission.[10] In Zimbabwe, the American Board Mission established a mission station at Mt. Selinda in 1893[11] and its legacy is still evident in the United Church of Christ in Zimbabwe and in its various schools and hospitals, including the first school founded at Mt. Selinda in 1893.[12] The American Board Mission also established another station at Chikore (Craigmore) 15 miles west of Mt. Selinda and had many satellite stations.[13] In Mozambique, the American Board Mission established stations at Beira in 1905 on the Indian Ocean coast and at Gogoyo in 1917, about 35 miles east of Mt. Selinda.[14]

These missions were established after extensive exploration and experimentation. As the American Board Mission expanded its work from South Africa, its first port of call was the Inhambane Bay in southeastern Mozambique where it opened a station in 1880. However, the mission's highest decision-making body, the Prudential Committee, voted to abandon the Inhambane site after 13 years of operation because of poor health conditions and sought to open a new site inland. After three expeditions to Gazaland, one in 1879 to Mzila, another in 1888 to Gungunyana, and the last one in 1891, the Prudential Committee authorized the "Pioneer Expedition to Gazaland" in May 1892. This expedition consisted of Rev.

[9] R. A. Shiels, "Aldin Grout (1803–1894), a founder of the American Zulu mission in Southern Africa," *Quarterly Bulletin of the South African Library*, 49, 4 (1995): 202. See also R. A. Shiels, "Early American Presbyterian missionaries in Southern Africa, Henry Isaac Venable 1834–1839 and Alexander Erwin Wilson 1834–1838," *Quarterly Bulletin of the South African Library* 50, 3 (1996): 140–151.

[10] J. Smith, *A History of the American Board Missions in Africa* (Boston, MA: American Board of Commissioners for Foreign Missions Congregational House, 1905), 28.

[11] Mount Selinda is modern name for Mount Silinda. It is an Anglicized version of Chirinda, the Ndau name for this area. In Zimbabwe, the ABCFM would come to be known simply as the "American Board Mission."

[12] American Board of Commissioners for Foreign Missions Archives, Houghton Library, Harvard University, Cambridge, MA, U.S.A. (hereafter ABCFM) 15.6 Box 1, Report of Sub-Committee accepted and adopted by the Prudential Committee, February 14, 1893.

[13] ABCFM, 15.4, vol. 23, Report of the East Central Africa Mission under the American Board of Commissioners for Foreign Missions, 1901.

[14] ABCFM, 15.4 vol. 32, First Annual Report of Gogoyo Mission Station, 1917.

G. A. Wilder of the Zulu Mission, and Rev. F. R. Bunker and Dr. W. L. Thompson of the East African Mission (Inhambane).[15]

Following several weeks of travels and inquiries, the "Pioneer Expedition to Gazaland" concluded that the most desirable place for the new station was in the territory of Chief Mapungwana, within the limits of the BSAC on the northern slope of Mt. Selinda. This site had an elevation of about 4000 feet above sea level, "with fertile soil, sweet water, and a goodly native population near at hand."[16] This was the same site that Cecil John Rhodes had recommended to these missionaries in 1891. The American Board Mission received a total of 15,000 morgen (about 37,500 acres) of land from the BSAC of which 6000 was at Mt. Selinda and the remainder at Chikore.[17]

At this time the boundary between Zimbabwe and Mozambique had not been defined. However, when the Boundary Commission completed its work later in 1899, the missionaries found that much of their land had fallen into Mozambican territory although their main site at Mt. Selinda remained in Zimbabwean territory. This prompted efforts to open another station in Mozambican territory because neither of the two administrations tolerated cross-border movements of Africans. Africans from Mozambique could not travel at will to attend school and have medical care at Mt. Selinda in Zimbabwe. In 1912 the American Board Mission investigated the feasibility of opening a new station in Mozambique.[18] They wished to establish a chain of stations linking Mt. Selinda and Beira. By 1917, after protracted correspondence with the Mozambique Company, American Board missionary, Dr. W. T. Lawrence, established a station at Gogoyo, where he also set up a school and a clinic.[19] Missionary staff frequently moved across the border between the two stations. The American Board Mission also established some outstations in the Save Valley and in Rusitu and Mutema in eastern Zimbabwe. The Save Valley outstations encompassed areas such as Kondo, Chibuwe, Chisumbanje,

[15] ABCFM, 15.6, Box 1, "Report of Sub-Committee accepted and adopted by the Prudential Committee," February 14, 1893.

[16] Ibid.

[17] ABCFM 15.4, volume 23, Report of East Central Africa Mission under the American Board of Commissioners for Foreign Missions—submitted by the Congregational Church of the United States and Canada, 1901.

[18] ABCFM 15.4, volume 32, Special Meeting of the Rhodesia Branch of American Board Mission in South Africa, Mt Silinda. October, 15–17, 1912.

[19] ABCFM 15.4, volume 32, "First Annual Report of Gogoyo Mission Station," 1917.

and Mahenye. Mt. Selinda remained the center of mission activities and it was the first to have a hospital, followed by Chikore.

Among other things, the missionaries hoped to erode the foundations of traditional society by creating a new class of individualist westernized Christians operating in the market economy.[20] Mission policy toward traditional medicine and traditional doctors was also influenced by the same strategy, with mission doctors considering traditional doctors to be institutional rivals and trying to undermine their influence by inculcating biomedical knowledge of disease. One major difference between state medicine and missionary medicine was that whereas state medicine emphasized an "ethnic model of collective pathology," mission medicine focused on individual Africans and individual accountability for sin and disease.[21] In the end, however, mission-educated Africans became some of the most vocal nationalists.[22]

Anglo-Portuguese Relations

Throughout the colonial period Rhodesians treated their Portuguese neighbors with contempt. They considered the Portuguese colonial state to be too weak to foster any meaningful development and therefore regarded Mozambique as a threat to the health of Zimbabwe.[23] The border therefore became a problem for colonial public health officials. Colonial authorities in Zimbabwe argued that the Mozambique Company

[20] Rennie, "Christianity, Colonialism and the Origins of Nationalism," 65.

[21] Vaughan, *Curing their Ills*, 57.

[22] For more on Christian missions and nationalism, see Rennie, "Christianity, Colonialism and the Origins of Nationalism," A. Helgesson, "Catholics and Protestants in a clash of interests in Southern Africa," in *Religion and Politics in Southern Africa*, ed. C. Hallenceutz and M. Palmberg (Uppsala: The Scandinavian Institute of African Studies: Seminar Proceedings, no. 24, 1991), 194–206, and Teresa Cruz e Silva, *Protestant Churches and the Formation of Political Consciousness in Southern Mozambique, 1930–1974* (Basel: P Schlettwein Publishing, 2001).

[23] For more on the Portuguese colonial administration, see Leroy Vail, "Mozambique's Chartered Companies: The Rule of the Feeble," *The Journal of African History* 17, 3 (1976): 389–416, Allen F. Isaacman and Barbara Isaacman, *Mozambique: From Colonialism to Revolution, 1900–1982* (Boulder, CO: Westview Press, 1983), and Elizabeth Lunstrum, "State Rationality, Development, and the Making of State Territory: From Colonial Extraction to Postcolonial Conservation in Southern Mozambique," in Christina Folke Ax, ed., *Cultivating The Colonies: Colonial States and Their Environmental Legacies* (Athens: Ohio University Press, 2011), 110.

government did not do enough to control diseases. Hence, they complained that diseases frequently spread from the Portuguese side of the border into Zimbabwe. However, the Portuguese also alleged that diseases were spreading into their territory from Zimbabwe and took preventive measures. These back and forth accusations and fears among colonial officials clearly demonstrate that the border was a major problem in the implementation of public health policy. Yet, while there were efforts to coordinate the control of livestock diseases, the same could not be said of human diseases.[24] This lack of cooperation was a departure from early attempts at cooperation in the colonial world, particularly in the pre-1914 period.[25]

Although it was true that the Mozambique Company did not have the same amount of resources that the BSAC had, it also embarked on coercive public health policies such as smallpox vaccinations. The scale of these public health initiatives was dictated by the availability of resources and the presence or absence of pressure from European settlers. In order to safeguard their own health, settlers pushed the colonial governments to embark on public health programs that were intrusive and discriminatory.

While all new settlers faced financial problems, the Colonial Zimbabwean Government quickly came to the rescue of its settlers by providing loans and other incentives to start commercial farming. However, lacking in funds, the Mozambique Company resorted to granting large sub-concessions to companies and individuals in return for a share of their profits. The financial problems of this company could be traced back to the beginning of its operations in the region, involving its failure to construct a railway from Manica to the coast. This was one of the fundamental requirements in the Mozambique Company's charter. While this railway was meant to provide communication essential to the development of mining, it was also probably influenced by the realization that Britain would not recognize Portugal's claims in East Africa unless it was guaranteed with ready access to the coast.[26] Without any means with which to

[24] For Anglo-Portuguese efforts to control livestock diseases, see Dube, "'In the Border Regions of the Territory of Rhodesia.'"

[25] Deborah Neill, *Networks in Tropical Medicine: Internationalism, Colonialism, and the Rise of a Medical Specialty, 1890–1930* (Palo Alto: Stanford University Press, 2012), 2–3. See also Maureen Malowany, "Unfinished Agendas: Writing the History of Medicine of Sub-Saharan Africa," *African Affairs* 99 (2000): 325–349.

[26] Barry Neil-Tomlinson, "The Mozambique Chartered Company, 1892 to 1910," 21.

construct the railway, the Mozambique Company conceded this right to a Dutch businessman, who after failing to raise the capital later conceded this right to the BSAC, which quickly formed the Beira Railway Company and built the railway. Thus, despite Portugal's anti-British sentiment during the scramble, it was finally the BSAC which built the railway from Mutare, Zimbabwe, to Beira, Mozambique.[27]

In this way then, Mozambique's colonial economy was dependent on neighboring colonial economies. Even the construction of the railroad infrastructure combined with forced labor, low pay, and poor working conditions, which forced many Africans to search for perceived better pay in the neighboring territories, served the interests of the neighboring British colonies more than those of Mozambique itself.[28] In fact, these British connections, British investment in the Mozambique Company, and Rhodesian influences gave the Mozambique Company's capital, Portuguese Beira, an English flavor, with English currency, English banks, an English press, English civil servants, and the widespread use of the English language.[29]

It was not long before the missionaries of the American Board Mission joined Rhodesians in condemning Portuguese colonialism. The missionaries perceived Portuguese colonialism as a threat to their religious goals and the health of the region in general. While they also condemned forced labor on settler farms in Zimbabwe, the American missionaries had a particularly low opinion of the morality of the Portuguese and considered the Portuguese colonial regime oppressive of Africans and of religious freedom. The American missionaries pushed to have Portugal stripped of her colonial possessions at the 1919 Paris Peace Conference. Their efforts failed, but these deliberations demonstrate the extent of their resentment of the disruption of African society by forced labor, slavery, and other colonial demands. They also reflect the perceived susceptibility of Mozambique (and Angola) to proposals for redivision in favor of "more economically developed colonial powers, that is, Britain and Germany, which continued to surface with some regularity until the 1930s."[30]

[27] Ibid., 30.

[28] Ndege, *Culture and Customs of Mozambique*, 15. The neighboring British colonies included South Africa, Zimbabwe, Malawi, and Zambia.

[29] Leon P. Spencer, *Toward an African Church in Mozambique: Kamba Simango and the Protestant Community in Manica and Sofala, 1892–1945* (Mzuzu: Mzuni Press, 2013), 26.

[30] David Hedges, introduction to *Protestant Churches and the Formation of Political Consciousness in Southern Mozambique, 1930–1974* (Basel: P Schlettwein Publishing, 2001), xii.

For their part, the Portuguese disliked Protestant missions such as the American Board Mission and the Swiss-Presbyterian Mission established in the 1880s in southern Mozambique. They disliked the use of English at Beira by the American missionaries. In general, however, after 1897, the Portuguese viewed the Protestant missions' continued emphasis on African languages, culture, and the reluctance to embrace or promote Portuguese culture as contradicting their post-conquest colonial goal of cultural and religious assimilation.[31] Portuguese antipathy toward and fear of Protestant missions were worsened by the perceived economic weakness of Mozambique, combined with the emergence of African nationalism in South Africa, fortified by Garveyism and African Trade Unionism in the 1920s.[32] It is worth noting that the first president of Mozambique's liberation movement Frente de Libertação de Moçambique (FRELIMO), Eduardo Mondlane, had been raised in the Protestant Swiss Mission Church in southern Mozambique.[33]

By the 1920s, therefore, the Portuguese considered Protestant missions in general as "'denationalizing' Mozambicans in the sense not only of 'detribalising' but also of facilitating assimilation to the more prestigious cultural alternatives available in and through South Africa and, to a lesser extent, Southern Rhodesia."[34] Thus when Antonio Salazar proclaimed the *Estado Novo* after the military coup in Portugal in May 1926, reclaiming Portuguese national agency in the colonies from largely English-speaking foreigners, as well as the closer integration of the Catholic Church with this objective, became the focus. This contributed to further tensions and the active discrimination against Protestant churches in the 1930s.[35] Protestant churches thus faced difficulties because of barriers imposed by the Portuguese.[36] The following section details cross-border movements that affected the epidemiology of diseases and

[31] Ibid.

[32] Ibid.

[33] G. Jan van Butselaar, "The Role of Churches in the Peace Process in Africa: The Case of Mozambique Compared," in *The Changing Face of Christianity: Africa, the West, and the World*, ed. Lamin Sanneh and Joel A. Carpenter (Oxford: Oxford University Press, 2005), 102.

[34] Hedges, introduction, xii–xiii.

[35] Ibid.

[36] Cruz e Silva, *Protestant Churches and the Formation of Political Consciousness*, 2. For a more in-depth discussion on the relationship between church and state in Portugal and its colonies, see G. Jan van Butselaar, "The Role of Churches in the Peace Process in Africa,"

contributed to the so-called denationalization of Portuguese colonial subjects.

Colonial Hardships: Land Alienation, Taxation, Forced Labor, Dipping Fees

As stated earlier, the establishment of the border was accompanied by a particularly virulent type of colonialism, full of discriminatory legislation, land alienation, taxation, forced labor (*chibharo*), and a myriad of fees that the colonial government demanded from Africans.[37] Robin Palmer noted that while Europeans seized African land everywhere in Zimbabwe, land alienation was more ruthless in two areas. One was in the land of the Ndebele (Matebeleland) in the western part of Zimbabwe, where the BSAC granted invading Europeans farms of 6350 acres, which were double the size of the Mashonaland farms, and the *high veld* on areas inhabited by the Ndau Ndebele.[38] In the lands of the Shona (Mashonaland), however, there was only one place that matched this extent of land expropriation and that was the district of Chipinge, where, following the evacuation of Gungunyana in 1889, the BSAC was eager to occupy the land before "natives ... come in and fill it up again."[39] Therefore, after the (T. Dunbar) Moodie Trek of 1892–1893, the BSAC authorized Europeans to peg off farms of 6350 acres in areas of dense Ndau population.[40]

As to the effects of this land alienation, Palmer argues that most Zimbabweans did not experience the immediate effects of the appropriation of 15.8 million acres because of the relatively small size of the African population, which was estimated to be around 750,000 in 1890, and also because only a few Europeans actually occupied and worked the farms which they had acquired on paper.[41] This meant that in many areas, Africans still had access to land which was now owned by Europeans. In Chipinge, however, Palmer notes that the African experience was quite

101–103, Spencer, *Toward an African Church in Mozambique*, 26, and Ndege, *Culture and Customs of Mozambique*, 23.

[37] For more on forced labor, see Charles Van Onselen, *Chibaro: African Mine Labour in Southern Rhodesia, 1900–1933* (London: Pluto Press, 1976).

[38] Palmer, *Land and Racial Domination in Rhodesia*, 38.

[39] Ibid., 41.

[40] Ibid. Dunbar Moodie named the area Melsetter after the town where he came from in Scotland.

[41] Ibid., 38–39.

different. This was one district where the Shona felt immediate land pressures, "for the rapacious Dunbar Moodie was nicknamed *Dabuyazizwe*, the one who divides the land, and such was his brutality that a report of 1895 revealed that 'the natives are running away from G. B. D. Moodie's farms as fast as they can.'"[42] All this prompted the local Native Commissioner (hereafter NC), T. B. Hulley, to call for the creation of a "native reserve" to settle Africans in the likely event of their being evicted from European farms in the future, and reduce the chances of an African uprising.[43] What differentiated Chipinge from Matabeleland, however, was the fact that Chipinge was occupied not by rich land speculators and miners but by poor Afrikaner farmers fleeing the agricultural depression in the Orange Free State of South Africa, and lured by promises of huge farms. Thus after the Moodie Trek, the Martin and Steyn Treks followed between 1893 and 1898, purposefully seizing areas densely settled by Africans for their fertility and resident labor.[44] This adversely affected Africans, as the settlers, lacking financial resources, thoroughly exploited African labor, including forcing Africans on European-owned farms to work for three months per year without pay.[45]

Apart from land alienation, there was a host of other immediate pressures on Africans, for example, forced labor and taxation, including the hut tax, first implemented in Mashonaland in 1894. This hut tax was ten shillings per hut and was collected in cash or kind.[46] Thus, this tax consisted of cash, or in grain, cattle, or even alluvial gold, or in labor, usually of two months' duration, with Africans being paid below market prices while exchanging their cattle for cash to pay the tax.[47] It is noteworthy that by 1895 the colonial government was averaging about £5000 per year in tax revenue and seizing as much as one-third of the Shona cattle, sheep, and goats in some districts, unleashing a systematic and brutal assault on the material wealth of the Shona.[48] Therefore, it is not surprising that the

[42] Ibid., 41.

[43] Ibid. Native Commissioners were members of the Native (African Affairs) Department responsible for representing African interests. They were some of the early critics of colonial state policies.

[44] Alexander, *The Unsettled Land*, 19.

[45] Palmer, *Land and Racial Domination in Rhodesia*, 90.

[46] Chengetai J. M. Zvobgo, *A History of Zimbabwe, 1890–2000 and Postscript, 2001–2008* (New Castle: Cambridge Scholars Publishing, 2009), 17.

[47] Palmer, *Land and Racial Domination in Rhodesia*, 44.

[48] Ibid.

Shona rose up in revolt in 1896, and although there was no revolt in Chipinge, this can be attributed to the lack of clear political authority after the Gaza evacuation and the fact that Chipinge had escaped the rinderpest cattle disease, which wiped out cattle in other districts.[49]

Meanwhile the land question never disappeared, with concerns over the provision of land for African use leading to the creation of "native reserves," following the South Africa precedent. As Palmer notes, the appearance of these reserves in Zimbabwe, and later in Kenya and Zambia, clearly demonstrated the devastating extent of alienation which had already taken place, because the reserves usually symbolized marginal land left over by Europeans.[50] Hence, a number of Africans ended up in reserves, others remained tenants on European-owned farms, still others lived on unalienated or "Crown" land, while a few who met the skill and capital requirements set by the colonial government could purchase freehold farms in precisely the same way as European settlers in African Purchase Areas.[51]

Yet matters were about to get worse for Africans, not as a result of the mineral revolution, as was the case in South Africa, but as a result of the failure to discover a "Second Rand." Hence, after their tour of Zimbabwe in 1907, the BSAC directors, influenced by developments in Kenya, decided to diversify the economy by encouraging European farming, with a "white agricultural policy" beginning in 1908, which radically altered the position of Africans on the land.[52] This was the case because in order to recover all the best land available, the colonial government launched an attack on the "native reserves" in the years 1908–1914. Then, with the reorganization of the Department of Agriculture in 1908, the government established a Land Bank to provide credit facilities to Europeans only and these services were not available to African farmers until 1945.[53]

However, this onslaught on African rights to land was not limited to the reserves. The position of Africans on both alienated and unalienated land was also reconsidered. It came to light that European farmers had been charging Africans rents ranging from 10 shillings and 40 shillings usually with an additional 10 shillings for each wife after the first, in a practice known as "Rack-renting," which the NCs hated because it was

[49] Ibid.
[50] Ibid., 57.
[51] Ibid., 61–62.
[52] Ibid., 80.
[53] Ibid., 81–82.

"immoral" and which "*bona fide* white farmers" hated too because it locked up both land and labor.[54] Thus in 1908, the government introduced the Private Locations Ordinance, modeled on Cape legislation, and aiming at limiting the numbers of Africans on European farms and penalizing absentee landlords, but its enforcement was delayed until 1920 due opposition from absentee landlords.

Yet the government's attack on African rights to land was unrelenting. In 1909 the BSAC imposed a rent on unalienated land, further contributing to the movement of Africans into the already shrinking and infertile reserves. There is evidence that the African inhabitants of Chipinge were hit the hardest. As Palmer noted, in Chipinge, the extensive land grab by Europeans coupled with total inadequacy of the reserves caused much hardship and resulted in all Africans targeted by the rents transferring their homes to reserves or alienated land.[55] Clearly, the inhabitants of the Zimbabwe-Mozambique border region under study bore the brunt of oppressive colonial policies. Another piece of oppressive legislation was the 1930 Land Apportionment Act, which, along with its successor, the 1969 Land Tenure Act, sealed the fate of African rights to land.

The loss of land was only one of the many oppressive practices of the colonial state. The state passed a myriad of discriminative legislation aimed at putting Africans at a disadvantage while simultaneously promoting the welfare of European settlers. In the 1930s, for example, after repeated outbreaks of foot-and-mouth disease on Nuanetsi and Devuli ranches in the southern part of Zimbabwe, the government selectively enforced quarantine regulations. It prohibited the movement of African-owned cattle (about 400,000 head) between and from reserves in the Ndanga, Chivi (Chibi), Gutu, Matobo, Chipinge, Masvingo (Victoria), and Bulilima-Mangwe districts for lengthy periods, while allowing white ranchers to carry on their business.[56] These restrictions boosted the cattle prices for white ranchers due to the removal of African-owned cattle from the national surplus and thus creating a captive market.

In similar fashion, as Ian Phimister concluded, the Maize Control Acts of 1931 and 1934 depressed prices paid to Africans in order to subsidize white farmers' return by employing "a complicated quota distribution

[54] Ibid., 89.

[55] Ibid., 96–97.

[56] Ian Phimister, *An Economic and Social History of Zimbabwe, 1890–1948: Capital Accumulation and Class Struggle* (London: Longman, 1988), 184–185.

which favoured whites, and a marketing system which discriminated against blacks."[57] Thus, while African farmers received an average price per bag ranging from 1 shilling and 6 pence to 6 shillings and 6 pence between 1934 and 1939, white farmers received an average price of over 8 shillings per bag during the same period. The net result of all of this was extreme suffering for most peasants and workers, engendered by a deliberate state policy of deflecting the Depression's main impact onto Africans and away from European settlers. Hence, "where jobs did not simply disappear, wages were reduced. Where access to land did not actually cease, markets were restricted, if not by the vagaries of capitalism, then by the exigencies of settler colonialism.'[58] In addition, African villagers also resented being forced to work on the construction of dipping tanks, which was largely aimed at protecting European settlers' exotic, disease-prone cattle. As Phimister noted, these developments, combined with the further erosion of chiefly authority and by the weakening of family bonds, contributed to economic distress and social dislocations, resulting in open antagonism toward the state.[59] Many villagers found solace in the message of preachers and indigenous prophets, including the *Vapostori* and Zion churches, as detailed in Chap. 6.

Yet the hardships for Zimbabwean villagers were not about to end any time soon. In 1951, the government introduced the Native Land Husbandry Act (NLHA), an act which further entrenched the state's agrarian control by forcing Africans to work on conservation projects in reserves, ostensibly to stem "overpopulation and resource degradation."[60] The real issue, however, was that the reserves had shrunk over the years as settlers claimed more land, and being situated in marginal areas, these reserves could not support the increasing African population. Yet, instead of giving Africans more land, the state sought to increase the carrying capacity of these reserves by embarking on dubious conservation projects such as the construction of storm drains and de-stocking. The government expected the NLHA to be a *dual spatial fix* that would bind peasants to rural reserves while requiring urban wageworkers to live in townships, entirely dependent on wage labor, now that they were cut off from subsistence production in the reserves.[61] Facing an increasingly ever oppressive

[57] Ibid., 185.
[58] Ibid., 196.
[59] Ibid., 196.
[60] Donald S. Moore, *Suffering for Territory: Race, Place, and Power in Zimbabwe* (Durham, Duke University Press, 2005), 83.
[61] Ibid., 83.

colonial state, Africans actively resisted these measures, leading to the suspension of the NLHA in 1962.

This NLHA had contradictions, just like many aspects of colonial rule. While creating an African workforce, residing permanently in urban areas, the state did not move fast to provide housing for married workers. In addition, as shown in the following chapter, migrant wage labor was what really powered the colonial economy, with translocal circuits of wage labor migration as Africans straddled footholds in smallholder agriculture and urban jobs. The effect of the NLHA's dual spatial fix would be the dislocation of routes and roots, as well as the disruption of translocal links and rural homesteads.[62]

Furthermore, demonstrating the importance of precolonial networks of interdependence in an area with much environmental diversity, the NLHA was even more problematic in the Zimbabwe-Mozambique border region. As Jocelyn Alexander correctly observed, in Chimanimani, the highveld Ngorima reserve's dense population and unusual ecology made the NLHA's need to simplify and categorize absurd because the area had never been centralized and no conservation measures or de-stocking had been implemented previously.[63] Worse still, due to Ngorima's interdependence with Mozambique and neighboring commercial farms, the NLHA's preoccupation with self-contained economic "units" was destined to fail. For then as now, families lived, farmed, and herded livestock on both sides of the Zimbabwe-Mozambique border, which voided the procedures for assessing carrying capacity. Moreover, because the majority of Chimanimani's chieftaincies had large followings in Mozambique and other districts, the NLHA's search for "functional communities" with clear boundaries was not viable.[64]

The story was not much different on the other side of the border in Mozambique, where Eric Allina has chronicled brutal forced labor practices akin to slavery under Mozambique Company rule.[65] Also, in some areas of Mozambique as in other parts of Africa, the colonial state forced Africans to cultivate cotton, impoverishing rural households.[66] As Allen and Barbara Isaacman have noted, the colonial state introduced a number

[62] Ibid., 85.

[63] Alexander, *The Unsettled Land*, 56.

[64] Ibid., 95.

[65] See, Allina, *Slavery By Any Other Name*.

[66] See Allen Isaacman, *Cotton is the Mother of Poverty: Peasants, Work, and Rural Struggle in Colonial Mozambique, 1938–1961* (Portsmouth, NH: Heinemann, 1996) and Allen

of tax laws designed to force many African agriculturists off their land and to create a pool of cheap labor for European plantations, for the embryonic light industrial sector, and for the port towns of Lourenço Marques and Beira.[67] They argue that many peasants were able to circumvent the labor requirement by cultivating new or additional cash crops to pay their taxes while others opted to work in the mines and plantations of neighboring South Africa and Zimbabwe at wages that were 200–300 percent higher than those in Mozambique. However, the forced labor code that had been first introduced in 1899, providing the legal rationale for forced labor, continued under varying forms until 1961. For example, in the 1930s, the Antonio Salazar regime, using the rhetoric of moral duty, passed legislation which obligated a majority of African men to work for six months or more as contract laborers, either for private employers or for the state, in order to pay their taxes.[68]

Thus, the pivotal element of Mozambique's colonial experience was the extraction of cheap labor through state intervention, including contract labor, the system of forced labor, the use of penal labor, and the labor supply treaties with South Africa and Zimbabwe, leading to the loss of hundreds of thousands of the most productive members of rural society. As a result of the departure of these workers, there was a restructuring of rural society, with reduced agricultural productivity, which was exacerbated by forced cotton and rice production, leading to increased debt, famines, disease, and soil erosion.[69] Africans therefore endured many hardships, which shaped their perception of the colonial state and its legitimacy, as well as public health.[70] These hardships were even more pronounced in a

Isaacman and Richard Roberts (eds.), *Cotton, Colonialism, and Social History in Sub-Saharan Africa* (Portsmouth, NH: Heinemann, 1995).

[67] Isaacman and Isaacman, *Mozambique*, 32.

[68] Ibid., 41.

[69] Ibid., 53. See also Lunstrum, "State Rationality, Development, and the Making of State Territory," 110.

[70] For more on the oppressive practices of the colonial state, see Sabelo J. Ndlovu-Gatsheni, "Mapping Cultural and Colonial Encounters, 1880s–1930s," in Brian Raftopoulos and A. S. Mlambo eds, *Becoming Zimbabwe: A History from the Pre-colonial Period to 2008* (Harare, Weaver Press, 2009), 64, A. S. Mlambo, "From the Second World War to UDI, 1940–1965," in Brian Raftopoulos and A. S. Mlambo eds, *Becoming Zimbabwe: A History from the Pre-colonial Period to 2008* (Harare, Weaver Press, 2009), 76, and Joseph Mtisi, Munyaradzi Nyankudya and Teresa Barnes, "Social and Economic Developments during the UDI Period," in Brian Raftopoulos and A. S. Mlambo eds, *Becoming Zimbabwe: A History from the Pre-colonial Period to 2008* (Harare, Weaver Press, 2009), 115–140.

border region, where the border interfered with villager's ability to access resources on the other side of the border, including health resources. The following chapter examines the responses of African villagers to colonial states' attempts to confine them within the colonial border.

References

Alexander, Jocelyn. *The Unsettled Land: State-making and the Politics of Land in Zimbabwe, 1893–2003.* Oxford: James Currey, 2006.

Allina, Eric. *Slavery By Any Other Name: African Life Under Company Rule in Colonial Mozambique.* Charlottesville: University of Virginia Press, 2012.

Allina-Pisano, Eric. "Negotiating Colonialism: Africans, the State, and the Market in Manica District, Mozambique, 1895–c. 1935." PhD Dissertation, Yale University, May 2002.

Cruz e Silva, Teresa. *Protestant Churches and the Formation of Political Consciousness in Southern Mozambique, 1930–1974.* Basel: P Schlettwein Publishing, 2001.

Dube, Francis. "'In the Border Regions of the Territory of Rhodesia, There Is the Greatest Scourge…': The Border and East Coast Fever Control in Central Mozambique and Eastern Zimbabwe, 1901–1942," *Journal of Southern African Studies* 41, 2 (2015): 219–235.

Hedges, David. Introduction to *Protestant Churches and the Formation of Political Consciousness in Southern Mozambique, 1930–1974.* Basel: P Schlettwein Publishing, 2001.

Helgesson, A. "Catholics and Protestants in a clash of interests in Southern Africa." In *Religion and Politics in Southern Africa*, edited by C. Hallenceutz and M. Palmberg. 194–206. Uppsala: The Scandinavian Institute of African Studies: Seminar Proceedings, no. 24, 1991.

Isaacman, Allen. *Cotton is the Mother of Poverty: Peasants, Work, and Rural Struggle in Colonial Mozambique, 1938–1961.* Portsmouth, NH: Heinemann, 1996.

Isaacman, Allen and Isaacman, Barbara. *Mozambique: From Colonialism to Revolution, 1900–1982.* Boulder: Westview Press, 1983.

Isaacman, Allen and Richard Roberts, ed. *Cotton, Colonialism, and Social History in Sub-Saharan Africa.* Portsmouth, NH: Heinemann, 1995.

Jan van Butselaar, G. "The Role of Churches in the Peace Process in Africa: The Case of Mozambique Compared." In *The Changing Face of Christianity: Africa, the West, and the World*, edited by Lamin Sanneh and Joel A. Carpenter. 97–115. Oxford: Oxford University Press, 2005.

Lunstrum, Elizabeth. "State Rationality, Development, and the Making of State Territory: From Colonial Extraction to Postcolonial Conservation in Southern Mozambique." In *Cultivating The Colonies: Colonial States and Their*

Environmental Legacies, edited by Christina Folke A. 107–121. Athens: Ohio University Press, 2011.
Malowany, Maureen. "Unfinished Agendas: Writing the History of Medicine of Sub-Saharan Africa." *African Affairs* 99 (2000): 325–349.
Maxfield, Charles A. "The Formation and Early History of the American Board of Commissioners for Foreign Missions." (2001). http://www.maxfieldbooks.com/ABCFM.html (14 September 2013).
Mlambo, A. S. "From the Second World War to UDI, 1940–1965." In *Becoming Zimbabwe: A History from the Pre-colonial Period to 2008*, edited by Brian Raftopoulos and A. S. Mlambo. 75–114. Harare, Weaver Press, 2009.
Moore, Donald S. *Suffering for Territory: Race, Place, and Power in Zimbabwe*. Durham, Duke University Press, 2005.
Mtisi, Joseph, Munyaradzi Nyankudya and Teresa Barnes. "Social and Economic Developments During the UDI Period." In *Becoming Zimbabwe: A History from the Pre-colonial Period to 2008*, edited by Brian Raftopoulos and A. S. Mlambo. 115–140. Harare, Weaver Press, 2009.
Ndege, George O. *Culture and Customs of Mozambique*. Westport, CT: Greenwood Press, 2007.
Ndlovu-Gatsheni, Sabelo J. "Mapping Cultural and Colonial Encounters, 1880s–1930s." In *Becoming Zimbabwe: A History from the Pre-colonial Period to 2008*, edited by Brian Raftopoulos and A. S. Mlambo. 39–74. Harare, Weaver Press, 2009.
Neil-Tomlinson, Barry. "The Mozambique Chartered Company, 1892 to 1910." PhD Thesis, School of Oriental and African Studies, University of London, 1987.
Palmer, Robin. *Land and Racial Domination in Rhodesia*. Berkeley: University of California Press, 1977.
Phimister, Ian. *An Economic and Social History of Zimbabwe, 1890–1948: Capital Accumulation and Class Struggle*. London: Longman, 1988.
Pophiwa, Nedson. "The Political and Economic Relations between Mozambique and Zimbabwe, 1890s to the Present: A Literature Review." Unpublished paper, Department of Economic History, University of Zimbabwe, 2005.
Rennie, John Keith. "Christianity, Colonialism and the Origins of Nationalism among the Ndau of Southern Rhodesia, 1890–1935." PhD Thesis, Department of History, Northwestern University, 1973.
Shiels, R. A. "Aldin Grout (1803–1894), A Founder of the American Zulu Mission in Southern Africa." *Quarterly Bulletin of the South African Library*, 49, 4 (1995): 202.
———. "Early American Presbyterian Missionaries in Southern Africa, Henry Isaac Venable 1834–1839 and Alexander Erwin Wilson 1834–1838." *Quarterly Bulletin of the South African Library* 50, 3 (1996): 140–151.

Smith, Judson. *A History of the American Board Missions in Africa*. Boston, MA: American Board of Commissioners for Foreign Missions Congregational House, 1905.

Spencer, Leon P. *Toward an African Church in Mozambique: Kamba Simango and the Protestant Community in Manica and Sofala, 1892–1945*. Mzuzu: Mzuni Press, 2013.

Vail, Leroy. "Mozambique's Chartered Companies: The Rule of the Feeble." *The Journal of African History* 17, 3 (1976): 389–416.

van Onselen, Charles. *Chibaro: African Mine Labour in Southern Rhodesia, 1900–1933*. London: Pluto Press, 1976.

Vaughan, Megan. *Curing Their Ills: Colonial Power and African Illness*. Stanford: Stanford University Press, 1993.

Zvobgo, Chengetai J. M. *A History of Zimbabwe, 1890–2000 and Postscript, 2001–2008*. New Castle: Cambridge Scholars Publishing, 2009.

CHAPTER 4

Colonial Border Restrictions and the African Response

The Border and Regional Population Movements

With the imposition of the border, the Ndau and Manyika chiefs found their land divided between the BSAC and the Mozambique Company. At the same time, colonial states began to restrict African mobility across the border to prevent the loss of labor, among other things. However, the Portuguese side of the border "hosted few white settlers and was ineffectively administered, leaving an important space for movement."[1] Some of the Shona of the border region therefore turned to labor migration, taking advantage of the porous Zimbabwe-Mozambique border. The extent of cross-border movements, which had important implications for the control of infectious and communicable diseases, is, therefore, the subject of this chapter.

As Jocelyn Alexander noted, in Chimanimani, the challenge for white farmers was controlling African labor, which was difficult because the burdens of tax and demands of farmers caused constant movement into remote areas of the mountains, into reserves, or across the border.[2] As a result, many white farmers in Zimbabwe were largely dependent on migrant labor from Malawi, Mozambique, and Zambia because the Shona preferred to farm on their own account.[3]

[1] Alexander, *The Unsettled Land*, 19.
[2] Ibid., 29.
[3] Palmer, *Land and Racial Domination*, 65.

F. Dube, *Public Health at the Border of Zimbabwe and Mozambique, 1890–1940*, African Histories and Modernities,
https://doi.org/10.1007/978-3-030-47535-2_4

Thus, as early as the 1890s, in their contestation of the border, villagers devised ways of resisting bureaucratic controls of the border. In the Manica district of Mozambique, for example, villagers devised a tax evasion strategy of fleeing to Zimbabwe, semi-permanently or permanently. Communities in Manica district were mobile. After all, these borderland people shared many cultural attributes with their Zimbabwean counterparts and were now being arbitrarily separated from friends and relatives by European-imposed borders. Hence, for Africans living close to the border, where the dangers of flight were minimal, people availed themselves of the border's permeability. These were people who had previously lived on or farmed land that now fell in British territory. In the same vein, many "Portuguese" Africans had "British" African relatives across the border. They also became aware that crossing the border relieved them from the tax and labor demands of the Mozambique Company government.[4] The same was true for Africans in the English territory.

Matters came to a head in 1907 when economic growth in Manica district strained the relationship between the Mozambique Company administration and the African population because of competition for African labor among rural African households, white employers, primarily farmers and miners, and the local administration.[5] Here, the predatory recruitment sweeps of African labor, often with the help or intervention of local chiefs, was ineffective because of the porous border.[6]

Farther south in Moribane after 150 conscripts returned from rubber collection work and revealed their wretched experience, several chiefs fled with all their subjects.[7] In other parts of the border region, for example, in the chiefdom of Machipanda, some Africans resided in Zimbabwe but had fields in Mozambique, thus paying the hut tax neither to the Portuguese nor to the English.[8] African villagers found ways of circumventing the border restrictions and labor and tax demands. In some cases an African chief would reside on one side of the border while his subjects were found on the other and several African men also sent their wives to settle on the opposite side of the border, while many others lacked a permanent abode

[4] Allina-Pisano, "Negotiating Colonialism," 91.

[5] Ibid., 123.

[6] Ibid.

[7] Allina, *Slavery By Any Other Name*, 92.

[8] Ibid. This practice is common in the border region, with people living in Mozambique planting fields in Zimbabwe.

on either side.[9] African villagers were well aware of the perceived economic weakness of Mozambique. As Portuguese officials recounted, African emigration to British territories was a triple blow, involving the loss of laborers, tax revenues, and irrefutable evidence of African preference for British rule, which was always a thorny issue among Portuguese nationalists.[10] In order to curtail African mobility, the Mozambique Company government resorted to extended "correctional" labor, beatings with the *palmatória* ("the perforated wooden paddle"), and deportation to São Tomé (off the West African coast), which hosted laborers from all corners of Portugal's far-flung empire laboring on cocoa plantations in what was tantamount to a life sentence.[11] Yet, as Portuguese officials admitted, border policing was a war they could not win because Africans who wanted to leave the territory usually avoided the roads.[12] As stated earlier, there was heavy demand for laborers in Zimbabwe. Colonial Zimbabwean statistics clearly demonstrate its reliance on Mozambican labor, for example, Mozambicans constituted 25.44 percent of the labor force in September 1906, 27.13 percent in December 1906, and 25.33 percent in March 1907.[13]

In their attempts to control cross-border movements, Portuguese officials required that Africans seek passes before crossing into Zimbabwe. Those who violated these laws were sentenced to up to 20 months of forced labor.[14] The data generated by these officials shows that only small numbers of Africans sought passes to Zimbabwe. Africans from Manica district usually visited border areas in Zimbabwe, such as Chipinge, Mutare, and Penhalonga. They went to trade, to visit relatives and friends, to buy household goods, and to seek medical attention. The most frequently visited places were Mutare, followed by Penhalonga, and then Chipinge. The areas in Zimbabwe visited by Africans from the Mossurize district were numerous, including Chipinge, Mt. Selinda, Jersey, Chikore, Mutema, Save, Mahenye, Muzite, Dondo, and Mapungwana. However,

[9] Ibid.

[10] Rhodesian officials, for instance, reported that the majority of Africans who applied at the Native Commissioner's office for certificates stated that "they have come from Portuguese territory and wish to live in British!" See NAZ, A3/18/20-22, W. Wood, Recruiter, Chipinga to C. W. Terry, Manager, Shamva, 30 June 1917.

[11] Allina, *Slavery By Any Other Name*, p. 95.

[12] Ibid., 96.

[13] Gelfand, *A Service to the Sick*, 45.

[14] Allina, *Slavery By Any Other Name*, 143.

the majority of Africans never bothered to seek permission to visit Zimbabwe as there were many clandestine entry points dotted all along the border.

On the other side of the border in Zimbabwe, the British were also having problems with Africans leaving for work in South Africa, where the entry level salary was 60 shillings and officials admitted, “It is a difficult problem for after all a native cannot be blamed for going where he can get most money.”[15] There were also regular movements into Mozambique to visit relatives and family and to trade goods.

Much of the movement across the border, however, remained lopsided, with Colonial Zimbabwean officials sometimes detecting huge influxes in Mozambican migrants. When the population of Chipinge district increased from 33,360 in 1922 to 36,568, the Chief Native Commissioner asked the Native Commissioner (NC) for that district to verify his figures and the NC “replied to the effect that they [figures] were in order and that what appeared to be an abnormal increase was chiefly due to the influx of natives from Portuguese territory.”[16] In 1924 the NC Mutare estimated the “alien floating population” at 4200 compared to 4150 in 1923.[17] He added that most of these aliens were resident in Mutare Township, on mines and railway compounds. Although that number of “aliens” included Africans from other territories, such as Malawi and Zambia, those from Mozambique constituted the greatest percentage, given its proximity to Mutare.

As a testimony to the existence of extensive cross-border movements, in 1924 the Mozambique Company administration launched an inquiry on the clandestine migration of Africans to South Africa and Zimbabwe and various *Chefes de Circunscriçãoes* (District Heads) provided estimates and the reasons for the emigration. The *Chefe* of Manica district estimated that about a hundred Africans emigrated annually and that these primarily went to Zimbabwe. The *Chefe* of Moribane, south of Manica, claimed that approximately 400 Africans migrated to South Africa and 200 to Zimbabwe yearly. Farther south, the *Chefe* of Mossurize estimated that about 1500

[15] NAZ, A3/18/20-22, W. Wood, Recruiter, Chipinga to C. W. Terry, Manager, Shamva, 30 June 1917.

[16] NAZ, S235/501 District Reports: Native Commissioners, Review of Reports of Native Commissioners Division III for the Year ended 31st December, 1923.

[17] NAZ, S235/502 District Reports: Native Commissioners, Report of the Native Commissioner, Umtali District, for the Year ended 31st December, 1924.

Africans migrated to Zimbabwe and South Africa annually.[18] These officials who were charged with border control probably gave low estimates which were wildly and deliberately inaccurate. They wanted to show that they were doing a good job of monitoring the border.

The reasons for this emigration were many and varied. The *Chefe* of Manica indicated the primary reason as the wish for better salaries which allowed them to quickly procure the bride price (*roora/lobola*). For the *Chefe* of Moribane, the main reason was "to obtain better salaries and good treatment," while the *Chefe* of Mossurize indicated that emigration was a "racial tradition," and added other reasons such as "better salaries, good treatment, and to get money for marriage (£25)."[19] In South Africa, Mozambican migrants usually worked on the Rand gold mines while in Zimbabwe, they labored in the agricultural as well as mining sectors.

Working on the Rand mines went beyond the pragmatic consideration of wages to include issues of gender and masculinity in African society. As the administrator of the Mozambique Company claimed in 1934, the African of Mossurize, "from boyhood, has only one ambition in life, which is to work for the Rand, and, as soon as he reaches the age of paying tax, he goes out in the path towards 'John' [Johannesburg or Joni], as they say, given that he who does not work in the mines in not considered a man."[20] One interviewee recalled how young men who had gone to Johannesburg (*Joni* in Shona) came back to take all the girls as they had money and were well respected.[21] It became difficult for men who stayed behind to compete for brides with labor migrants returning from South Africa.

The story was the same for the border communities of Zimbabwe, where young men of Chimanimani considered labor migration to South Africa as the status of a "custom," with migrants even using false names and Portuguese addresses to migrate illegally.[22] Thus, work in South Africa

[18] Arquivo Histórico de Moçambique, Maputo (hereafter AHM), Fundo da Companhia de Moçambique (hereafter FCM), Secretaria Geral (SG), Repartição do Gabinete-Processos, 1903–1942, Inquérito sobre a emigração clandestine para o Transval e Rodésia, 1924, Caixa 76, I-35. For an extensive discussion of the labor migration to Rhodesia, see Joel das Neves, *O trabalho Migratório de Moçambique para a Rodésia do Sul, 1913–1958/60* (Maputo: Universidade Pedagógica, 1990).

[19] Ibid.

[20] Hughes, *From Enslavement to Environmentalism*, 36.

[21] Interview, Harare, Zimbabwe, 10 July, 2006.

[22] Alexander, *The Unsettled Land*, 29.

was an important lifeline for both Mozambicans and Zimbabweans of the border region, contributing to extensive cross-border movements.

On the question of how "better" were the salaries from Zimbabwe and Transvaal for Mozambicans, the *Chefe* of Moribane indicated that Africans who migrated to Zimbabwe were paid £1 and those who went to the Transvaal obtained up to £5 per month.[23] By some estimates, the average wage of African labor migrants in South Africa was £3 per month, substantially more than the average African wage in either Mozambique or Zimbabwe.[24] Work in the mines and plantations of South Africa and Zimbabwe paid wages that were more than double those offered by local Portuguese settlers. Similar disparities drove a considerable number of northern Mozambicans to the cotton and tea estates of Nyasaland and the sisal plantations of Tanganyika.[25]

While the official numbers of migrants cited above appear to be insignificant, there was extensive movement from Mozambique into Zimbabwe. The registered numbers were small because border monitoring was ineffective, at least in these early years of colonial rule, up to the 1920s. This weak control of the border could be one reason why the Colonial Zimbabwean settler community feared mobile Africans as sources of disease. These fears were heightened by the view among most settlers and Colonial Zimbabwean officials that Portuguese East Africa was a hotbed of disease and that Portuguese officials were not doing enough to combat disease. The Colonial Zimbabwean settlers therefore knew that the number of migrants was considerable, but they also knew that their government exerted little control over African movement.

As a result, cross-border movements continued. In 1925 the NC Mutare reported that 637 Africans from the Portuguese Territory had acquired domicile in the district, while that for Melsetter sub-district reported that a few Africans from Portuguese Territory had settled on the Crown lands and farms in the eastern part of the sub-district as well as in the Ngorima reserve.[26] In 1926 the NC Chipinge reported that 168

[23] AHM, FCM, SG, Repartição do Gabinete-Processos, 1903–1942, Inquérito sobre a emigração clandestine para o Transval e Rodésia, 1924, Caixa 76, I-35.

[24] Rennie, "Christianity, Colonialism and the Origins of Nationalism," 198.

[25] Allen Isaacman, "Coercion, Paternalism and the Labour process: The Mozambican cotton regime 1938–1961," *Journal of Southern African Studies* 18, no. 3 (1992): 486–526.

[26] NAZ, S235/502 District Reports: Native Commissioners, Report of the Native Commissioner, Umtali District and Melsetter sub-District, for the Year ended 31st December, 1925. "Crown Land" was land not yet apportioned, thus considered to belong to the Queen.

African men, some of them with families, came to live in the district from adjoining Portuguese Territory whereas the NC Chimanimani reported that several Africans went to live in Portuguese Territory, returning "whence they came a few years ago."[27] This suggests that there was enough movement across borders to alter the disease environment in the region, either by reducing the amount of labor available for environmental modification or through the spread of infections.

That cross-border movements were common was also shown by the increase in applications from Mozambique for permission to reside in Zimbabwe. For instance, the NC Mutare reported in 1929 that Africans from the neighboring districts of Portuguese Territory frequently applied for permission to become domiciled in Zimbabwe. This permission was granted only "after careful investigation" of whether land was available for them and of their previous history.[28]

However, this movement was not always one way. Africans in Zimbabwe also frequently crossed the border into the Portuguese territory for various reasons. In 1929, for instance, nine adult Africans moved to the Portuguese Territory.[29] Similarly, when drought struck in Zimbabwe in 1933, the NC Chipinge reported that, driven by famine, which was general throughout the district south of Chipinge, large numbers of Africans wandered away into adjoining Portuguese Territory in search of food so that, at times, certain areas appeared to be almost depopulated.[30]

Moreover, while the *Chefe* of Mossurize reported that approximately 403 Africans were working in Zimbabwe and the Transvaal in 1937,[31] the NC Chipinge reported in 1938 that the failure of crops due to drought made it difficult for Africans to procure sufficient food to sustain them until the next season and, as a result, many of them traveled miles into the

[27] NAZ, S235/504 District Reports: Native Commissioners, Report of the Native Commissioner, Melsetter District and Melsetter sub-District, for the Year ended 31st December, 1926.

[28] NAZ, S235/507 District Reports: Native Commissioners, Report of the Native Commissioner, Umtali District, for the Year ended 31st December, 1929.

[29] Ibid.

[30] NAZ, S235/511 Volume III: Native Commissioners Reports, Report of the Native Commissioner for the Melsetter District for the Year ended 31st December, 1933.

[31] AHM, FCM, Negocios Indigenas-Processos, Caixa 26, Pasta 166-Trabalho Indigena-Diversos Assuntos, O Chefe de Mossurize para Exmo. Senhor, Diretor dos Negocios Indigenas, Beira, 15 April 1937.

adjoining Portuguese Territory to barter grain from their more fortunate neighbors.[32]

Apart from these border crossings in times of crisis, Africans from both sides of the border always mingled for a variety of reasons. Applications to domicile in Zimbabwe continued to pour in from Mozambique for various reasons. Some applicants were discontented with the conditions of life in Portuguese Territory, while others stated that all their surviving relations were in Zimbabwe and another group comprised those who had lived in Zimbabwe for many years and had married indigenous wives. However, the NC Mutare indicated that owing to the "extremely limited space available," in the Mutare district for African settlement, these applications were only "granted in exceptional circumstances."[33] The 1930s and 1940s also witnessed sharp increases in the number of Mozambicans entering and residing in Mutare district. For instance, the number of "Portuguese Africans" as a proportion of the Colonial Zimbabwean labor force in the Mutare district increased from 21.1 percent in 1931 to 25.4 percent in 1936 and from 43.0 percent in 1941 to 51.1 percent in 1946.[34]

Despite border surveillance efforts, movements across the border continued. In 1947 the Clerk in charge of the Native Department at Penhalonga reported that 449 Africans from Mozambique migrated to the district, but he had also issued 115 passes to Africans from Mozambique to leave Zimbabwe.[35] These are only a few documented cases of cross-border movements. There was much more "clandestine" movement across the border. For example, the NC Chipinge claimed that because the majority of Africans employed on farms along the border areas were from

[32] NAZ, S235/516 District Reports: Native Commissioners, Report of the Native Commissioner, Chipinga, for the Year ended 31st December, 1938.

[33] NAZ, S235/516 District Reports: Native Commissioners, Report of the Native Commissioner, Umtali, for the Year ended 31st December, 1938. While claims of insufficient land were reasonable, the strong demand for migrant Portuguese African labor contributed to denials of permission to settle in Rhodesia. Rhodesian officials feared that if Portuguese migrants settled in the colony, they soon would shun the farms and mines just like the local villagers and result in labor shortages.

[34] Richard Hodder-Williams, *White Farmers in Rhodesia, 1890–1965: A history of the Marandellas District* (London: Macmillan, 1983), 166.

[35] NAZ, S1051 Native Commissioners Reports: Report of the Clerk in charge, Native Department, Penhalonga, for the quarter ended 31st December, 1947.

Mozambique, they were "liable to disappear over the border when they tire of work."[36]

As an indication of the extent of movement and colonial Zimbabwe's dependence on Mozambique for labor, a 1961 Chipinge district annual report lamented the shortage of labor as a result of a new Employment Act.[37] This Act was supposed to discourage the employment of Africans from Portuguese East Africa and the vacuum thus created was to be filled by indigenous Africans from reserves and towns. However, due to labor shortages, Colonial Zimbabwean employers in the border areas voiced the opinion that this Employment Act had not achieved its purpose, although still acknowledging that the Act had not been in operation sufficiently long enough to assess its worth. In order to make this Act work, the employers pressed for a brake on immigration from Portuguese East Africa, the introduction of a quota system, and limiting the number of registration certificates issued each month by the pass offices.

The developments of the mid-1970s, however, further complicated cross-border mobility. After gaining its independence under the leadership of the Mozambique Liberation Front (Frente de Libertação de Moçambique or FRELIMO), socialist and anti-colonial Mozambique found itself surrounded by hostile neighbors, Southern Rhodesia, at that time led by Ian Smith's fascist, white-supremacist government, and apartheid South Africa. These colonial governments became concerned when FRELIMO actively supported African nationalist movements in both countries, leading to a campaign of destabilization in Mozambique by providing support to groups of Mozambicans who were disillusioned with FRELIMO and who eventually organized under the name Resistência Nacional Moçambicana (RENAMO/Mozambican National Resistance). Elizabeth Lunstrum notes that although RENAMO had some measure of political legitimacy, particularly in the center of the country, "in the rest of the country it functioned primarily through an economy of terror and violence, working not so much to put in place a new political leadership, but to destroy Frelimo and what it had accomplished."[38] This general

[36] NAZ, S2827/2/2/3 Native Commissioners Reports: Annual Report for the Year ended 31st December, 1955. Native Commissioner, Melsetter.

[37] NAZ S2827/2/2/8 Annual District Report, Melsetter, 1961, vol. II.

[38] Lunstrum, "State Rationality, Development, and the Making of State Territory," 115. See also Margaret Hall and Tom Young. *Confronting Leviathan: Mozambique Since Independence* (Athens: Ohio University Press, 1997), Malyn Newitt, *A History of Mozambique*, Alex Vines, *Renamo: Terrorism in Mozambique* (Bloomington: Indiana

instability, including the raging war of independence in Zimbabwe and counter-insurgency measures by the settler government made border crossing hazardous, particularly for Africans who could not obtain passes to cross the border and who ended up using undesignated entry points. Therefore, many Mozambicans lost limbs and lives while trying to cross the mine-infested border in the 1970s in search of food after drought and famine struck their lands. Some interviewees recounted the ordeal in this way,

> After independence in Mozambique [1975], there were shortages of basic commodities such as salt, soap and cloth. The only alternative was to cross the border into Rhodesia. But at this time, the war of independence had begun in Rhodesia. People started to go and steal from the settlers in Rhodesia. Then the Rhodesians planted land mines. Many people perished from these mines as they attempted to procure salt and soap. There was a general lack of hygiene due to these shortages and people resorted to using leaves of wild plants and chaff [by-product of pounding maize corn] as soap. These methods were not very effective in removing dirt. It was impossible to wash blankets. So, people shaved their heads [to get rid of lice] and wore sacks. The only people who wore clothes were those who had husbands or fathers working in South Africa, but even for them it was not easy to get these clothes because goods from South Africa now had to come through Maputo, not by the easier route through Rhodesia. Maputo was too far [more than 1,000 kilometers or more than 621 miles] and most of the bridges along the way had been destroyed or closed. So, the closure of the [Zimbabwe-Mozambique] border caused much pain and suffering.[39]

Movements across the border thus continued, even during these perilous times. What this demonstrates is that the border between Mozambique

University Press, 1991), and Ken Wilson, "Cults of Violence and Counter-Violence in Mozambique," *Journal of Southern African Studies* 18 (1992): 527–582.

[39] Group interview, Chambuta, Mozambique, 22 September 2006. Many interviewees in Mozambique cited the problems they encountered while attempting to cross the border. After the Zimbabwean war of independence (Second Chimurenga) commenced in the 1970s, the colonial government planted landmines along the Zimbabwe-Mozambique border to prevent the movement of Africans to and from training camps in Mozambique (had just gained its independence in 1975). The colonial government closely monitored the official entry points to the extent that Mozambicans who were facing famine could not easily cross to get food from Zimbabwe. They therefore resorted to using the mine-infested bush paths. Many interviewees indicated that they knew of the dangers but there was no alternative. Many domestic and wild animals were also caught up in these mine-infested areas.

and Zimbabwe was permeable. It was this permeability which heightened the fears of the threat of disease transmission from one colony to another, particularly from the supposedly poorly governed Mozambique Company territory.

Conclusion

As stated earlier, the physical, political, economic, and social aspects of the Zimbabwe-Mozambique border region, before and during colonial rule, are important in assessing the ecological changes in the region as a result of the imposition of colonial rule and the resultant transformation in disease ecologies, which is the subject of Chap. 5.

One major part of the discussion has been the African response to the colonial border. It is clear, therefore, that the extensive cross-border movements, which were reinforced by colonial labor demands, heightened fears of disease transmission. As a result, colonial authorities set up border surveillance to control the movement of Africans and their livestock across the border. However, this monitoring of the border caused much hardship as African villagers were forced by circumstances to use treacherous bush paths. As the following chapter shows, restrictions on the movements of Africans and livestock across the border due to trypanosomiasis interfered with precolonial patterns of transhumance and led to the disruption of life in African communities. What all this shows, however, is that the border, contested as such by Africans, became a public health problem for the colonial governments.

References

Alexander, Jocelyn. *The Unsettled Land: State-making and the Politics of Land in Zimbabwe, 1893–2003.* Oxford: James Currey, 2006.

Allina, Eric. *Slavery By Any Other Name: African Life Under Company Rule in Colonial Mozambique.* Charlottesville: University of Virginia Press, 2012.

Allina-Pisano, Eric. "Negotiating Colonialism: Africans, the State, and the Market in Manica District, Mozambique, 1895–c. 1935." PhD Dissertation, Yale University, May 2002.

Gelfand, Michael. *A Service to the Sick: A History of the Health Services for Africans in Southern Rhodesia, 1890–1953.* Gwelo: Mambo Press, 1976.

Hall, Margaret and Tom Young. *Confronting Leviathan: Mozambique Since Independence.* Athens: Ohio University Press, 1997.

Hodder-Williams, Richard. *White Farmers in Rhodesia, 1890–1965: A history of the Marandellas District*. London: Macmillan, 1983.

Hughes, David. M. *From Enslavement to Environmentalism: Politics on a Southern African Frontier*. Seattle: University of Washington Press in association with Weaver Press, Harare, 2006.

Isaacman, Allen. "Coercion, Paternalism and the Labour process: The Mozambican Cotton Regime 1938–1961." *Journal of Southern African Studies* 18, 3 (1992): 486–526.

Lunstrum, Elizabeth. "State Rationality, Development, and the Making of State Territory: From Colonial Extraction to Postcolonial Conservation in Southern Mozambique." In *Cultivating The Colonies: Colonial States and Their Environmental Legacies*, edited by Christina Folke A. 107–121. Athens: Ohio University Press, 2011.

Newitt, Malyn. *A History of Mozambique*. Bloomington: Indiana University Press, 1995.

Palmer, Robin. *Land and Racial Domination in Rhodesia*. Berkeley: University of California Press, 1977.

Rennie, John Keith. "Christianity, Colonialism and the Origins of Nationalism among the Ndau of Southern Rhodesia, 1890–1935." PhD Thesis, Department of History, Northwestern University, 1973.

Wilson, Ken. "Cults of Violence and Counter-Violence in Mozambique." *Journal of Southern African Studies* 18 (1992): 527–582.

PART III

The Border and Public Health

CHAPTER 5

The Political Ecology of Disease Control: The Border and Sleeping Sickness

Trypanosomiasis has received a great deal of attention from scholars. As Maureen Malowany, correctly observed, what is unique about the history of medicine in Africa has been the inter-relationships of environment and disease, public health and biomedical care, with human disease challenges, particularly in epidemic form, intimately linked to ecological changes.[1] The first authoritative works to address the environmental dimension of trypanosomiasis control are C. F. M. Swynnerton's "Examination of the Tsetse Problem in North Mossurise, Portuguese East Africa"[2] and John Ford's *The Role of African Trypanosomiases.*[3] These works basically examined the methods of environmental modification that Africans had used to control the disease before the establishment of colonialism. Building upon these works, this chapter considers the implication of the Zimbabwe-Mozambique border for the control of trypanosomiasis, particularly cooperation across the border, mainly to protect European-owned cattle. The border thus became productive in the implementation of disease control policies as a result of fears of the spread of the disease from Mozambique

[1] Malowany, "Unfinished Agendas," 330.

[2] Swynnerton, "Examination of the tsetse problem in North Mossurise, Portuguese East Africa."

[3] Ford, *The Role of African Trypanosomiases*. See also Helge Kjekshus, *Ecology Control and Economic Development in East African History: The case of Tanganyika 1850–1950* (Heinemann, London, 1977).

F. Dube, *Public Health at the Border of Zimbabwe and Mozambique, 1890–1940*, African Histories and Modernities,
https://doi.org/10.1007/978-3-030-47535-2_5

into Zimbabwe, with the British in Zimbabwe, arguing that Portuguese authorities were not doing enough to control the disease.

This trans-colonial cooperation was unique because for the most part trypanosomiasis control methods were restricted to colonial boundaries. Heather Bell has shown, for example, how British trypanosomiasis control initiatives in Sudan involved erecting barriers between infected areas, particularly adjoining francophone colonies, and uninfected zones and between humans and tsetse flies.[4] The only trans-colonial cooperation that existed was on scientific aspects, such as research and international conferences. Daniel R. Headrick has documented, for instance, how the Belgians in the Congo followed the recommendations of the Liverpool School of Tropical Medicine in 1903–1905 to implement stringent measures.[5] These measures included imposing *cordon sanitaires* around fly-infested areas and controlling the movement of people by requiring medical passports for travelers. The Belgian Congo's government then opened up camps for the sick, staffed by Catholic nuns, where Africans were diagnosed by palpating their neck glands, with those suspected of being infected quarantined in camps guarded by soldiers and injected with atoxyl. This was before the shift to decentralized ambulatory care, where itinerant teams examined villagers and medical corps opened rural clinics, hospitals, and injection centers.

While this level of cooperation was common in the Zimbabwe-Mozambique border, the perceived weakness of the Mozambique Company government and general Lusophobia among the British spawned fears of diffusion of disease, leading to the adoption of extra measures. Thus, while the Portuguese succeeded in eliminating trypanosomiasis on their little colony of Principe between 1922 and the 1950s using a blend of British, Belgian, and French methods, when it came to its larger colonies, Angola and Mozambique, neither the Portuguese government nor the colonial authorities possessed the money or manpower to contain outbreaks.[6] The methods employed in Principe included the clearing of undergrowth near human habitation; draining of swamps; cutting down trees; using workers wearing black cloths to attract, catch, and kill the tsetse flies; hunting and killing wild pigs, civet cats, monkeys, and stray

[4] See Bell, *Frontiers of Medicine in the Anglo-Egyptian Sudan*, 127–162.

[5] Daniel R. Headrick, "Sleeping Sickness Epidemics and Colonial Responses in East and Central Africa, 1900–1940," *PLOS Neglected Tropical Diseases* 8, 4 (2014): 4.

[6] *Ibid.*, 6.

dogs; examining and injecting people with atoxyl; segregating the sick in special camps; relocation of villages from infested areas; and closely monitoring the inhabitants. The result was that the proportion of inhabitants with trypanosomes in their blood dropped from 26 percent in 1907 to 0.64 percent in 1914.[7]

Yet, in the bigger colonies, controlling sleeping sickness was difficult, partly due to the conditions engendered by colonial rule itself. As colonial powers began to assert their authority after 1890, the demands of colonial economies and ineffective public health interventions led to the outbreaks of diseases in epidemic form. Little wonder that by the early twentieth century, many Africans understood the increased incidence of disease "as a kind of biological warfare" which accompanied conquest and establishment of colonial rule.[8] African means of controlling sleeping sickness through environmental modification became difficult to implement after the establishment of colonial rule. The nature of colonial economies therefore led to changes in disease ecologies in many parts of Africa.[9] Colonialism sought to exploit African land, mineral wealth, and labor. Heavy taxation and labor migration, whether "voluntary" or forced, greatly increased African mobility as colonial officials pressured Africans to work on mines and farms (especially in South Africa, Zimbabwe, and Kenya), to collect natural products such as rubber in the Belgian Congo, and to produce cash crops. Colonial officials also alienated African lands, beginning the process of "proletarianization" in settler colonies, such as South Africa, Zimbabwe, Kenya, and Algeria.

As the epidemics broke out, European colonial governments employed various strategies to control the disease. British East Africa, for instance, employed a largely environmental approach, which entailed separating humans from tsetse flies.[10] In Uganda, for example, where devastating

[7] *Ibid.*

[8] Maryinez Lyons, *The Colonial Disease: A Social History of Sleeping Sickness in Northern Zaire, 1900–1940* (Cambridge: University of Cambridge Press, 1992), 3.

[9] Meredith Turshen. *The Political Ecology of Disease in Tanzania* (New Brunswick: Rutgers University Press, 1984); Lyons, *The Colonial Disease*; Rita Headrick, ed., *Colonialism, Health and Illness in French Equatorial Africa, 1885–1935* (Atlanta: African Studies Association Press, 1994); and James Giblin, "Integrating the history of Land use into Epidemiology: Settler agriculture as the cause of disease in Zimbabwe," Working Paper No. 176 presented as part of the History of Land Use in Africa project of the African Studies Center, Boston University, and the Forest History Society, 1994.

[10] See Headrick, "Sleeping Sickness Epidemics and Colonial Responses," 4, M. Worboys, "The Comparative History of Sleeping Sickness in East and Central Africa, 1900–1914,"

epidemics were recorded in the early 1900s, Kirk Arden Hoppe has shown that the threat that sleeping sickness epidemics posed to the availability of African labor led the designation of certain environments as "Infected Areas," making human occupation in these areas illegal.[11] There were some important differences with Zimbabwe, however, perhaps stemming from the fact that Zimbabwe never had sleeping sickness epidemics such as those of Uganda, but the fear of Ugandan-type epidemics influenced sleeping sickness control policies. Thus, in the Mozambique-Mozambique border region, colonial governments forced Africans and their cattle to form buffer zones to protect white settlers. The crucial difference was, therefore, on how the economies were organized, with settler farming in Zimbabwe and Mozambique, and peasant farming in Uganda. Hoppe also found that for purposes of policing, communication, and commerce, British officials commenced the clearing of tsetse-harboring bush from a limited number of authorized roads and landings to allow essential human access through fly-infested land. However, in the Zimbabwe-Mozambique border region, vegetation clearing was implemented supposedly to prevent the spread of tsetse flies from Mozambique.

In general, the rhetoric of disease control became a convenient way for colonial governments to consolidate their authority over Africans through social engineering. For the Belgian Congo, where colonialism increased the mobility of people and pathogens and where sleeping sickness spread along rivers, the approach was largely medical. As Maryinez Lyons has shown, instead of attempting to separate humans from flies, the Belgian authorities focused on killing the trypanosomes in sick Africans in order to prevent their transmission.[12] As many scholars have noted, in the Belgian Congo, epidemic control provided a rationale for social control, showing the linkage between the interests of capital development and subservience to the colonial state.[13] Daniel Headrick has correctly observed that while the Belgian Congo won praise from Europeans for offering the "most effective and comprehensive medical care in any European colony," with

Hist Sci 32 (1994): 89–98, and Kirk Arden Hoppe, "Lords of the Fly: Colonial Visions and Revisions of African Sleeping-Sickness Environments on Ugandan Lake Victoria, 1906–61," *Africa* 67, 1 (1997): 86–105.

[11] Hoppe, "Lords of the Fly," 86–87.

[12] Lyons, *The Colonial Disease*, pp. 8–24; 34–35; 64–76; 102–141, See also Headrick, "Sleeping Sickness Epidemics and Colonial Responses."

[13] Malowany, "Unfinished Agendas," 331. See also Lyons, *The Colonial Disease*, Hoppe, "Lords of the Fly."

the Belgians themselves boasting about their health care system as proof of their civilizing mission, for Africans, "it meant living in a police state, with a health care system that only overcame an epidemic that European colonial rule had exacerbated in the first place."[14]

It can therefore be argued that the subsequent colonial efforts to control sleeping sickness were intended to correct the disease situation that had been worsened by the imposition of colonialism in the first place. In the Zimbabwe-Mozambique border region, these efforts included attempts to curtail the mobility of Africans and their livestock, rampant destruction of vegetation and wildlife, and use of chemicals. Although built upon African ideas of environmental modification, colonial wholesale destruction of flora and fauna did not fit well into the ecological setting. It also largely failed to produce the desired results, partly due to contradictions within colonialism. This chapter therefore deals with the increased incidence of sleeping sickness as a result of environmental change engendered by the imposition of colonial rule and cross-border movements of wildlife, as well as African villagers and their cattle. This contributed to colonial attempts to restrict the mobility of African cattle keepers across the border, particularly after 1900 as the much hoped for gold wealth did not materialize and the colonial states emphasized agriculture and cattle ranching as the mainstays of the economy. Demonstrating the centrality of colonial economies, this chapter also shows how these two colonies cooperated across the border to control animal trypanosomiasis, which was a threat to livestock.[15]

Many precolonial African societies, including those of Southern Africa, maintained control over trypanosomiasis through environmental modification, for example, through clearing vegetation in order to grow crops and through hunting.[16] Outbreaks of trypanosomiasis depended upon the ecological relationship between vectors, hosts, human populations, and the habitat. With the advent of colonialism, however, Africans lost control

[14] Headrick, "Sleeping Sickness Epidemics and Colonial Responses."

[15] The Rhodesian and Portuguese governments also cooperated to control East Coast Fever, which affected cattle, see Francis Dube, "'In the Border Regions of the Territory of Rhodesia, There Is the Greatest Scourge …': The Border and East Coast Fever Control in Central Mozambique and Eastern Zimbabwe, 1901–1942," *Journal of Southern African Studies* 41, 2 (2015): 219–235.

[16] For a more detailed examination of precolonial hunting patterns, see Clapperton Chakanetsa Mavhunga, *Transient Workspaces: Technologies of Everyday Innovation in Zimbabwe* (Cambridge, MA: MIT Press, 2014).

over the environment due to land alienation and other colonial demands, such as demands for wage and forced labor. Colonial rule in both Zimbabwe and Mozambique introduced new land-use patterns and labor requirements which affected the relationship between villagers and their environment and, in turn, altered their ability to control trypanosomiasis. In addition, the abandonment and neglect of land by European settlers and companies due to undercapitalization and for speculative purposes promoted the development of habitats which favored the growth of vector populations, leading to an increase in the incidence of trypanosomiasis outbreaks during the colonial period. The net effect of this was that colonial states, particularly Rhodesia, implemented invasive trypanosomiasis control measures which contributed to distrust of public health not only because they wanted to control bovine trypanosomiasis but also due to fear of spread of human trypanosomiasis. Yet this fear was based on an erroneous epidemiological understanding of trypanosomiasis. This mistaken thinking was influenced by Colonial Zimbabwean settlers' imagination of the border through a contemptuous feeling that Mozambique was a backward, poorly governed (by Iberians), and unhealthy territory.

This emphasis on diffusion of trypanosomiasis from Mozambique led European settlers in Zimbabwe to overlook the ecological changes (neglect and abandonment of land) engendered by colonialism within Zimbabwe itself which contributed to increase of trypanosomiasis in Zimbabwe. The fears of diffusion therefore served in a sense as a cover for the European settlers, allowing them to stir up fear of the spread of disease from the outside as a way of diverting attention from the neglect of land in Zimbabwe itself. Thus, the increase of trypanosomiasis cases in Zimbabwe involved two factors, one being the spread from Mozambique, but the other being changes in land use which made increased tsetse fly habitat in Zimbabwe.

Due to the fact that the border influenced settler imagination, colonial attempts to monitor cross-border movements in order to control trypanosomiasis led to the disruption of precolonial Shona networks of interdependence. Writing in 1971, an authority in both animal and human trypanosomiasis, John Ford, commented that the "existence of a modern international boundary on one side of which no development is taking place [Mozambique] suggests that it [trypanosomiasis] may continue to exist for many years to come."[17] Hence, the colonial border had a profound effect on efforts to control trypanosomiasis.

In their mission to eradicate "ignorance" and institute benefits of "civilization," the European colonists, on the surface, dismissed African knowledge systems as "primitive" and unscientific. They set aside much of the praise that early explorers gave to African agricultural systems in order to make way for colonial "science." Yet, behind the scenes, these colonial officials appropriated some of this knowledge as a key foundation of their programs beyond the rhetoric of primitivism. As was the case with other diseases, European settlers blamed Africans for the spread of trypanosomiasis. They perceived Africans as the reservoirs of infection and considered African migrants to be responsible for spreading infection. Africans, therefore, bore the brunt of erroneous and ineffective tsetse and trypanosomiasis control measures. Colonial land alienation pushed Africans to the marginal and tsetse-infested areas where they and their cattle became buffers between tsetse areas and white farms. The border also interfered with African grazing patterns and African mobility. Trypanosomiasis control measures involving cattle and game fences along the border prevented some forms of transhumance which had contributed to protecting cattle from trypanosomiasis in the precolonial period. However, trypanosomiasis was also intimately linked to environmental factors, such as rainfall, temperature, and vegetation, which made its control particularly challenging.

Trypanosomiasis is a vector-borne parasitic disease caused by *Trypanosoma*, which are protozoa transmitted to humans and animals by the tsetse fly (*Glossina*). It affects both humans and animals. In Zimbabwe and Mozambique, animal trypanosomiasis occurred wherever tsetse flies were prevalent. These tsetse flies exist widely in Africa and are usually found in vegetation along rivers and lakes, in gallery forests, and in vast expanses of woodland savannah.

Human African trypanosomiasis is also known as sleeping sickness. It is transmitted to humans by bites of tsetse fly which have acquired their infection from human beings or from animals harboring the human pathogenic parasites. Sleeping sickness exists in two forms. One is *Trypanosoma brucei gambiense* which occurs in Central and West Africa. This form has a long latency period, meaning that a person can be infected for several months or years without showing any symptoms of the disease. The

[17] Ford, *The Role of African Trypanosomiases*, 335.

symptoms emerge when the disease is already at an advanced stage. The second form is *Trypanosoma brucei rhodesiense* found in Southern and East Africa.[18] This form causes acute infection that emerges a few weeks after the tsetse fly bite. It tends to be more virulent than the former. As a result, it is detected earlier than the former strain. This strain is conveyed by tsetse fly *Glossina (G.) morsitans*, which infested northwestern parts of Zimbabwe and much of Mozambique, including the areas on the border with Zimbabwe.

The fact that the second strain of the disease was spread by *G. morsitans* is crucial because over the course of the colonial period, colonial officials in Zimbabwe invested much effort in trying to prevent the spread of *G. morsitans* from Mozambique in order to protect both domestic animals and humans.[19] Equally crucial was the belief in early twentieth-century Zimbabwe in the possibility of the transmission of a human trypanosome from a domestic animal. Researchers in Zimbabwe discovered around 1910 that some trypanosomes which could infect humans existed in both man and animals wherever *G. morsitans* were known to be present, and because at that time (1910) this type of fly was known to exist in over 10,000 square miles of Zimbabwe, the situation was alarming.[20]

Although there were no epidemics of human trypanosomiasis during the colonial period in the Zimbabwe-Mozambique border region, officials were still concerned about potential epidemics. As the Medical Director for Zimbabwe put it, in any district where the *Glossina morsitans* fly was common, there was always a grave possibility of an epidemic of sleeping sickness in the event of an outbreak being started by infective Africans.[21] This explains the high level of interest that the Colonial Zimbabwean Government invested in prevention and control methods in the Chipinge

[18] NAZ, S1173.266: Public Health Department—Human Trypanosomiasis, Southern Rhodesia, 1934. Rhodesian officials often indicated that this name was somewhat a misnomer (with the potential to hurt Rhodesian efforts to attract European settlers) as this strain occurred in other colonies, such as Tanganyika, Nyasaland, and Portuguese East Africa as well as in Northern and Southern Rhodesia.

[19] NAZ, F122/FH/30/1/1: The fight against tsetse fly in the British African Dependencies, undated (probably written in the period after 1955 because it quotes documents written that year).

[20] NAZ, S246/256: Notes on the Human Trypanosomiasis of Southern Rhodesia, undated (probably written in the period after 1934).

[21] NAZ, S1173/336: Preliminary Report on the Medical Treatment of Natives, R.A. Askins, Medical Director, Rhodesia, 8th September, 1930.

district, bordering portions of Mozambique that were infested with *G. morsitans*.

Embryonic research and erroneous views at that time also fanned the fears of epidemics. While some researchers thought that the animal trypanosome could not infect humans because of the trypanocidal action of the human blood, others believed that under certain conditions (pathogenic or dietetic), the trypanocidal substance disappeared from the human blood leading to susceptibility to infection with animal trypanosome.[22] However, the realization that both humans and animals were involved in the transmission of human trypanosomiasis amplified the public health threat posed by trypanosomiasis and subsequent colonial efforts to control human and animal (domestic and wild) mobility both within and across territorial boundaries.

As mentioned earlier, efforts to control trypanosomiasis were complicated by mobility across the inter-territorial boundary and by ecological transformations under colonial rule. The border was a factor because it divided a region whose environment was conducive to the prevalence of *Glossina*. In order to fully grasp the impact of trypanosomiasis control on the African reception of public health, it is necessary to examine the prevalence of trypanosomiasis in domesticated and wild animals partly because fears of the spread of human trypanosomiasis based on erroneous ideas affected public health policies, border monitoring, and, ultimately, African reception of colonial public health.

An example of erroneous ideas about trypanosomiasis was the claim by a Colonial Zimbabwean Veterinary official, E. W. Bevan, who asserted in 1934 that trypanosomiasis could be “transmitted by blood-sucking flies other than the tsetse, [making] the danger [posed by trypanosomiasis] … immeasurably greater.”[23] Bevan claimed that trypanosomiasis had been known to occur where the tsetse fly appeared absent. Entomologists were thus inclined to attribute these cases of trypanosomiasis to “mechanical transmission” by flies other than the tsetse. However, the current understanding of the transmission of the disease points to the tsetse fly as the only vector involved.

[22] NAZ, S246/256: Notes on the Human Trypanosomiasis of Rhodesia, undated (probably written in the period after 1934).

[23] NAZ, S246/524–525: Research in Trypanosomiasis, quarterly report by E.W. Bevan, Southern Rhodesia, 10th December, 1934. Bevan was a researcher in trypanosomiasis and his work was funded by the Beit Railway Trustees of London.

What happened under colonial rule can be classified into three processes: first, the partitioning of land and demands for labor which interfered with precolonial tsetse and trypanosomiasis control; second, the attempt by colonial officials to establish sterile zones around settlers' lands to prevent transmission; and third, the implementation of widespread eradication of flora and fauna in addition to border control methods and, from the 1950s onward, the use of drugs and residual insecticides to control the disease. Officials involved in tsetse and trypanosomiasis control efforts were from various departments, such as Veterinary, Public Health, Entomology, Native Affairs, Agriculture, and Tsetse Fly and Trypanosomiasis Control and Reclamation. In order to fully grasp the significance of environmental modification by precolonial societies and the colonial onslaught on flora and fauna, it is important to examine the roles of both vegetation and wildlife in the occurrence of trypanosomiasis.

The Ecology of Trypanosomiasis

Tsetse fly distribution is greatly influenced by environmental factors like density and type of vegetation and temperature. These factors, in turn, influenced tsetse control methods employed by colonial officials. Research on tsetse flies has shown their restriction to forests, woodlands, and tree savanna as an adaptation to avoid the perilous consequences of overheating and desiccation.[24] In 1942, R. W. Jack, former Chief Entomologist in Zimbabwe's Department of Agriculture, found, through laboratory experiments, that the loss of water was the most serious risk for tsetse flies, making this the greatest weakness in their life economy.[25] Temperature is also closely associated with altitude. In Zimbabwe, with a total area of 150,344 square miles, tsetse flies were not found in areas above 4000 feet above sea level. This reduced the potential area of infection to 100,000 square miles.[26] However, because Mozambique had more land below 4000 feet, the susceptible area was much larger there than in Zimbabwe.

Researchers believe that tsetse flies need shade, probably to shield them from excessive dehydration. The availability of trees is thus important for

[24] Ford. *The role of the trypanosomiases*, 288.

[25] R. W. Jack, "The Life Economy of a Tsetse Fly," *The Rhodesia Agricultural Journal*, 41 no. 1/2 (1944), 28.

[26] NAZ, S246/524–525: Research in Trypanosomiasis, quarterly report by E.W. Bevan, Southern Rhodesia, 10th December, 1934.

providing shade for tsetse flies. Grasslands do not support tsetse flies, but all forms of woodland, from savannah to rainforest, usually provide a suitable habitat for some species of tsetse flies. Artificially planted vegetation also provides a suitable habitat for tsetse flies and so too do thickets which develop on abandoned agricultural land, especially those comprising *Lantana camara* (Tickberry).[27] This plant existed in certain areas of the Chipinge district in Zimbabwe. In 1955 the NC for this district reported that *Lantana camara*, "a perennial decorative shrub, initially a garden escape, abounds in the Chinyaduma Division where it has ruined much valuable land."[28] Hence, tsetse flies need a conducive habitat in order to flourish.

Tsetse fly distribution was also dependent on the ecology of the fly. In Zimbabwe there were three species of tsetse, *G. morsitans*, *G. pallidipes*, and *G. brevipalpis*. *G. morsitans* existed in the rather dry northern part of the country, in and adjoining the Zambezi Valley, and was found again just across the southeastern border of the country. The two other species existed mostly in the wetter areas of Zimbabwe along a small part of the southeastern border near Mt. Selinda.[29] These two species were also present in high density on the Portuguese side of the border, as was *G. morsitans* and *G. austeni*. Colonial Zimbabwe's Chief Entomologist, R.W. Jack, noted that *G. morsitans* was an open forest tsetse fly, which avoided the interior of thickets and closed forests.[30] It was capable of enduring a comparatively dry, almost semi-arid climate, and it was apparently intolerant of humid conditions. That was why this species of tsetse occurred in the drier and less forested parts of Mozambique, while it was generally absent on densely forested and humid side of the border in Zimbabwe.

G. pallidipes and *G. brevipalpis*, by contrast, were dependent on thickets, and both could inhabit dense forest and humid zones, although *G. pallidipes* was not necessarily confined to such conditions. This explains why these two species occurred in the wetter and densely forested eastern

[27] R. J. Phelps and D. F. Lovemore, "Vectors: Tsetse flies," in *Infectious Diseases of Livestock, with Special Reference to Southern Africa*. Volume I, ed. J. A. W. Coetzer, et al. (Cape Town: Oxford University Press, 1994), 25–51.

[28] NAZ, S2827/2/2/3: Report of the Native Commissioner, Chipinga, for the year ending 31st December, 1955.

[29] NAZ, 483/53/2: Trypanosomiasis and Tsetse fly, 1948–1950—Meeting of the Technical Officers engaged on Tsetse fly control, 15th May 1950, Central African Council.

[30] NAZ, R.W. Jack, "The Tsetse fly problem in Southern Rhodesia," Reprinted from *Rhodesia Agricultural Journal*, Bulletin No. 892, May, 1933, 2.

highlands of Chipinge district, whereas *G. morsitans* was largely confined to the drier and less forested areas. Most southern parts of the Zimbabwe-Mozambique border region were heavily wooded, with a rainforest at Mt. Selinda extending into the Spugabera area of Mozambique. The Budzi River and its tributary, for instance, had "very dense patches of bush with a clearly defined double canopy" and more scattered patches of extensive forest in other areas, which could support *G. brevipalpis* and *G. pallidipes*, respectively, in summer months.[31]

In addition, the Rusitu River valley, which was "very densely wooded where untouched" by cultivation, provided habitat for *G. pallidipes* and perhaps *G. morsitans* as well.[32] The situation was the same on the eastern bank of the Save River (Sabi Division) in the southwestern part of Chipinge district, which was infested with *G. morsitans*, as were the Honde and Rupembi catchment areas and the Msaswe River. These caused a serious animal trypanosomiasis outbreak in the Musikavanhu reserve in 1954. The Makossa Hill located in this area, with predominant *Brachystegia tamarindoides* vegetation also harbored *G. morsitans*.[33] The NC Chipinge argued in 1958 that the control of the tsetse fly was made "extremely difficult by the dense bush and undergrowth and by the wooded ravines which pocket the Eastern Border," and felt that Tsetse control officials were losing the battle against the fly on the Chipinge front.[34]

The existence of *G. pallidipes* and *brevipalpis* on the Portuguese side of the border was also due to favorable ecological conditions. C. F. M. Swynnerton observed that there was "primary forest" consisting of "lofty, densely growing trees" that supported many woody lianas and lower tiers of evergreen shrubs with a "carpet and fringe" that could not

[31] NAZ, F122/400/7/35/3: Report on visit to the border clearing, by R.J. Phelps, Entomologist, Department of Tsetse and Trypanosomiasis and Reclamation, Southern Rhodesia, 24th April, 1958.

[32] NAZ, F122/400/7/35/3: Report on visit to the border clearing, by R.J. Phelps, Entomologist, Department of Tsetse and Trypanosomiasis and Reclamation, Southern Rhodesia, 24th April, 1958. The Rusitu River, located north of the border clearing, runs through the Chief Ngorima's area, the area that used to be called the Ngorima reserve before 1980. One of the dipping tank areas in this reserve, Ndima, recorded a number of trypanosomiasis cases in the 1950s.

[33] NAZ, FH122/400/7/35/2: Report of the Acting Director of the Department of Tsetse and Trypanosomiasis and Reclamation, Southern Rhodesia, 1956, 8.

[34] NAZ, S2827/2/2/6: Report of the Native Commissioner, Chipinga for the year ending 31st December, 1958.

readily burn.[35] He also noted that "primary forest" of the "rainforest" type existed in the highlands, mostly in small patches at Spungabera and in the Rusitu-Sitatonga rubber country. The trees that covered much of these rainforests were *Khaya nyasica* (East African mahogany or *mubaba*), *Chrysophyllum fulvum* (large *Muchanja*), and *Piptadenia buchanani* (*Umfomoti*). The *Muchanja* and *Umfomoti* trees largely dominated forest in the Rusitu-Sitatonga rubber country, giving it the characteristic of being regularly deciduous. However, the lianas and evergreen shrubs ensured the availability of shade for the forest fly, *G. brevipalpis*, and conditions conducive to its activities throughout the day.[36]

Swynnerton also noted the presence of "secondary forest," including the highly deciduous types (such as *Pterocarpus sericeus/Mubhungu*, *Pterocarpus angolensis/*Bloodwood or *Mubvangazi*) which harbored tsetse fly during the rainy season. He also recorded the presence of lowland bush savanna, *Brachstegia* wooding also known as *Tondo* bush or *Gusu*, dense secondary forest, and *Bauhinia* and *Erythroxylon-Landolphia* thickets. Among these, *Brachstegia* wooding was tsetse bush *par excellence*.[37] The distribution of sub-species of tsetse fly in Mozambique thus reflected the importance of vegetation in tsetse fly ecology. *G. austeni mossurizensis* was found in *miombo* woodlands with dense undergrowth in the high rainfall, medium- to high-altitude areas along the Zimbabwe-Mozambique border, while *G. austeni* was usually found in the drier coastal thickets.[38]

Apart from climatic factors, wild animals also played a major role in the occurrence of tsetse flies and trypanosomiasis in the border region. Many species of game, such as antelopes, African buffalo, warthog, and hippopotamus, were capable of surviving in tsetse fly areas.[39] These animals "sometimes have high infection rates of various *Trypanosoma* spp. and

[35] C. F. M. Swynnerton, "Examination of the tsetse problem in North Mossurise, Portuguese East Africa," 319.

[36] *Ibid.*, 320–321.

[37] *Ibid.*, 321.

[38] *Ibid.*, 37.

[39] R. D. Bigalke, "The important role of wildlife in the occurrence of livestock diseases in Southern Africa," in *Infectious Diseases of Livestock, with Special Reference to Southern Africa*. Volume I, ed. J. A. W. Coetzer, et al. (Cape Town: Oxford University Press, 1994). 155–163.

hence serve as excellent maintenance (reservoir) hosts for nagana [animal trypanosomiasis]."[40]

The tsetse flies also depended principally on wild animals for their blood meals, without which they could not survive. Thus, the distribution and abundance of some tsetse fly species, particularly *G. morsitans* and *pallidipes*, often referred to as the "game tsetse flies," were heavily reliant on the numbers and habits of certain wild animals.[41] That is due to the fact that tsetse flies prefer certain animals for their blood meals such as the warthog, and bushpig, as well as some bovidae like the kudu and bushbuck. However, tsetse flies also feed on the elephant, black rhinoceros, and African buffalo. The existence of these hosts therefore contributed to the maintenance of a tsetse fly population and the potential for trypanosomiasis.

Reflecting the importance of wild animals in the existence of tsetse, the rinderpest (cattle plague) epidemic which killed many wild animals, such as the buffalo, kudu, eland, bushbuck, bushpig, and warthog in the last quarter of the nineteenth century, led to the temporary disappearance of the fly.[42] This epidemic did not affect the region uniformly, however. In some localities, considerable numbers of wildlife and tsetse flies survived.

Tsetse and Trypanosomiasis Control Before Colonial Rule

An examination of precolonial tsetse fly and trypanosomiasis control methods shows that these methods were relatively more effective and environmentally friendly than subsequent colonial disease-control mechanisms. Studies of trypanosomiasis have shown that precolonial African societies successfully co-existed with trypanosomiasis as they achieved protection against the disease by modifying their environment in ways which affected the "sizes of and interaction among the five populations involved in the transmission of trypanosomiasis—humans, their livestock, wild

[40] R. D. Bigalke, "The important role of wildlife in the occurrence of livestock diseases in Southern Africa," 155.

[41] R. J. Phelps and D. F. Lovemore, "Vectors: Tsetse flies," 29.

[42] *Ibid.* Following this pandemic, tsetse flies disappeared from many areas demonstrating that the susceptible animals were their preferred hosts although nobody made this connection during that time. In fact, many observers thought the Rinderpest virus itself was pathogenic to tsetse flies, a theory which recent research has proved incorrect.

fauna, tsetse flies and the trypanosome parasites."[43] Villagers managed to achieve this not through wholesale eradication of tsetse flies and their habitats but through ensuring minimum but constant human and animal contact with pathogens. They controlled tsetse populations by altering its habitats through burning and clearing for fresh pastures, agriculture, and settlement. As trypanosomiasis researcher E. W. Bevan noted, in protozoal diseases such as trypanosomiasis, immunity tended to die out unless maintained by constant re-infection.[44]

In 1918 C. F. M. Swynnerton studied the methods of Mzila (son of the Nguni general, Soshangana) in controlling trypanosomiasis in the southern part of the Zimbabwe-Mozambique border region (Chipinge and Mossurize districts). Swynnerton noted that when Mzila came back from southern Mozambique to the Mossurize River valley in 1861 (an area that had been depopulated in 1831 by Zwangendaba during the *Mfecane*), he found that this area, previously occupied by a cattle-keeping agricultural community before Zwangendaba's invasion in 1831, was now covered with tsetse-infested woodlands.[45]

While Mzila set about capturing cattle from survivors of the Rozvi Empire, he could not reintroduce the cattle into the Mossurize valley in Mozambique, where his capital was located, because of trypanosomiasis. He kept these cattle on the mountain grasslands north of Chipinge. After several attempts to reintroduce cattle into the Mossurize River valley failed, Mzila ordered an "immense compulsory movement of the population. ... The bush simply disappeared and the country became bare, except for the numberless native villages and a continuity of native gardens," wrote Swynnerton.[46] Tsetse flies therefore disappeared from most settled areas because of this modification of the environment, but Mzila left some areas unsettled as wildlife reserves, particularly between the Sitatonga hills and the Budzi River which Swynnerton called the "Oblong." Swynnerton concluded that there was still plenty of tsetse in the *Brachstegia* wooding

[43] James Giblin, "Trypanosomiasis control in African history: An Evaded Issue?," *Journal of African History* 31, no. 1 (1990): 59–80. See also Ford. *The Role of the Trypanosomiases.*

[44] NAZ, S246/524–525: Research in Trypanosomiasis, quarterly report by E.W. Bevan, Southern Rhodesia, 10th December, 1934.

[45] Ford. *The Role of the Trypanosomiases,* 333. This area is called Mossurize or Mossurise in Mozambique. In Zimbabwe, it is called Musirizwi, all stemming from the Musirizwi/Mossurize River.

[46] Swynnerton, "An examination of the tsetse fly problem in North Mossurise, Portuguese East Africa," 332–333.

and that the fly never disappeared from the "Oblong." Thus, cattle could not be kept in these areas. The same applied to Chief Mtobe's area and the eastern part of Mafuse's chiefdom, close to the rubber forest.

Swynnerton also observed while progressing eastward across the Rusitu River of the rubber forests, that cattle could not be kept in this area, although Usele and other Zulu who settled there had made an attempt.[47] The cattle these "Zulu" (Shangani) needed for ceremonial purposes had to be brought from "safe" areas. Cattle could not be kept south of the Budzi either, from the Mwangezi eastward. These were the areas that were scarcely touched by Mzila's operations. Swynnerton argued that Mzila's tsetse operations never fully cleared the areas of chiefs Mtobe and Mafuse. He also observed that the rubber trees spread, offering a suitable habitat for tsetse flies, during the reign of Mzila's successor, Gungunyana, under encouragement from the Shangani who traded rubber for cloth on the Indian Ocean coast. These Shangani then used the cloth to barter for cattle in the border region.

However, in the cleared areas cattle-keeping succeeded. These areas included the Zinyumbo's hills on the Mwangezi, and westward through the Mossurize valley and northward to Spungabera. The same applied to the Gogoyo-Makuyana tract, where cattle were kept right under the Sitatongas, and on the Save River in Zimbabwe. Swynnerton's interviewees said that Chief Zinyumbo's area, like Chief Gogoyo's, was completely cleared, meaning that right up to the Mwangezi, it was gardens only, as was Chief Gwenzi's area, the Mossurise valley, and portions of the Save River.[48] When these areas were closely settled, cattle were kept successfully where they had failed before, although herds close to the tsetse areas suffered small and occasional losses.[49]

Swynnerton's account shows that villagers, unlike colonial officials, did not embark on wholesale vegetation and wildlife destruction in order to control trypanosomiasis. Instead, precolonial trypanosomiasis control was closely connected with land-use patterns which permitted occasional transmission of the disease from wildlife to cattle and maintained the disease in an endemic state with less mortality. Trypanosomiasis in this area was thus suppressed by settlement, before 1830 by the Rozvi Empire (which succeeded the Mutapa state) and again by Mzila after 1861.

[47] *Ibid.*, 333.
[48] *Ibid.*, 333.
[49] *Ibid.*, 334.

As Swynnerton suggested, the waxing and waning of the tsetse fly population in the border region between 1861 and 1889 resulted from changes in human population densities. The fact that this region was tsetse infested by 1861 can also be explained by the depopulation caused by Zwangendaba's massacres in the 1830s. Many "old people" had told Swynnerton's interviewees that prior to Zwangendaba's massacres, the people of this region successfully kept cattle, even to as far as the Sitatongas, where these "old people" had shown the interviewees some old cattle pits.[50] Chiefs Mafuse and Mtobe also told Swynnerton that cattle were kept in all parts of the colony where subsequent efforts to keep them had failed. Yet by the time Mzila arrived in Mossurize, the entire country had reverted to woodland and game had increased. "It was much as it is now," wrote Swynnerton in 1921, "fly had become plentiful, and the mountains of the present political border were the boundary, then as now, between the fly and such cattle as existed."[51]

Due to the rinderpest epidemic at the end of the nineteenth century, tsetse disappeared from the previously infested southern part of Zimbabwe and almost completely from the northern part, remaining only in a few small isolated "residual foci." From these residual foci tsetse began to spread, re-occupying their former natural haunts.[52] These residual foci included the heavily forested areas of the Zimbabwe-Mozambique border region, such as the "Oblong" and the Rusitu rubber plantations, from which the fly began to spread westward to the border area.

Colonialism only made the trypanosomiasis situation worse than it was in the precolonial period, leading to numerous outbreaks in cattle. This was partly a result of the fact that the colonial boundary interfered with long-standing forms of transhumance. These forms of transhumance involved movements of cattle from the low lands on the Mozambican side of the border to the highlands in Zimbabwe during the rainy season when the incidence of trypanosomiasis increased. The rains promoted the growth of lush vegetation and created humid conditions in the lowlands, thereby expanding the tsetse habitat. For instance, Mzila, kept his cattle on the grass-covered Chipinge highlands to protect them from

[50] *Ibid.*, 332.

[51] *Ibid.*

[52] NAZ, S483/53/2 Trypanosomiasis and Tsetse fly, 1948–1950: Coleman, Secretary to the Prime Minister, to the Chief Secretary, Central African Council, Salisbury, 14th April, 1950.

trypanosomiasis until he embarked on environmental modification to rid the Mossurize valley of tsetse flies.

The restrictions on cattle movements were a result of the cattle and game fences erected by tsetse and trypanosomiasis control officials as a trypanosomiasis control measure. This included the construction of a six-mile fence along a section of the border which was under the American Board Mission's area.[53] The missionaries indicated that the colonial government in Zimbabwe furnished the fence, but the cost of construction of this fence was met by the mission. In other parts of the border region the border fence was much longer. The NC Chipinge, for example, complained that although the clearing of bush on the Anglo-Portuguese border continued, it was unfortunate that considerable sections of the approximate 20 miles of fencing on the 55 miles stretch from the Rusitu River to international beacon 96 were damaged, possibly due to "clandestine" movement of stock and Africans.[54] Mr. T. Mbekwa from Mpanyeya, Mozambique, recalled, "the restrictions on the movement of cattle were a heavy blow to us because we were used to moving cattle from one place to another in search of fresh pasture and water."[55] While useful in finding fresh pastures, these movements also protected cattle from trypanosomiasis, but the colonial boundary restricted these practices. Hence the analysis now focuses on the changes in the epidemiology of trypanosomiasis brought about by colonialism.

Epidemiological Consequences of the Establishment of Colonial Rule

There is evidence that outbreaks of trypanosomiasis occurred as a result of the establishment of colonialism in the Zimbabwe-Mozambique border region. With the changes in land-use patterns in the colonial period, villagers lost control over the environment, which meant they also lost control over trypanosomiasis. As a result, the colonial assault on the environment and wildlife replaced precolonial practices as major means of controlling diseases.

[53] ABC 15.6, Volumes 8–11, Minutes of Mission Meetings, 1940–44: Semi-Annual Meeting of the East African Mission of the American Board, December 28th, 1939.

[54] NAZ S2827/2/2/3: Report of the Native Commissioner, Chipinga for the year ending 31st December, 1955.

[55] Interview with Mr. T. Mbekwa, Mpanyeya, Mozambique, 14 December, 2006.

Colonial land-use patterns made trypanosomiasis control more difficult. The introduction of new techniques of land management and pest control, as well as private ownership of land, worsened the trypanosomiasis situation and shifted the burden of trypanosomiasis control measures onto African villagers.[56] Colonial officials pushed Africans and their cattle to the unproductive and often heavily tsetse-infested areas, for example, the Musikavanhu and Ngorima reserves, which were prone to tsetse fly invasions. In this way Africans and their cattle provided a buffer zone between settlers and their cattle provided an indispensable buffer against the spread of the disease to European farms.[57]

With the establishment of colonialism, Africans lost their rights to land. The BSAC, for instance, considered land to be a commercial asset, to be sold to European settlers on easy terms.[58] Yet much of the alienated land, like the so-called Crown Land, was not actually under use. Most settlers also did not utilize all of their land either. Large tracts of land fell into the hands of absentee landlords and land speculators, leading to ecological problems and increased difficulty in controlling the tsetse fly and trypanosomiasis.

On the Zimbabwean side of the border region, particularly where the Shangani once settled (Gazaland), colonization was a family business for the Moodie family, who parceled out large tracts of land to their family members with the approval of Cecil John Rhodes.[59] This effort was led by Dunbar Moodie who pegged huge claims of land for himself, for his family, and for South African land and mineral speculators in the last quarter of the nineteenth century. An idea of the scale of these concessions can be gleaned from the fact that in order to encourage white settlement in this part of Zimbabwe, Rhodes was persuaded to give Gazaland settlers double the normal land allocation of 3000 acres per family.[60]

[56] Ford, *The Role of the Trypanosomiases*, 353.

[57] *Ibid.*, 354.

[58] The British South Africa Company led by Cecil John Rhodes acquired a royal charter from the Queen of England to colonize Mashonaland and Matebeleland, areas that form present-day Zimbabwe. The Company exemplifies the British method of establishing colonialism through chartered companies. It ruled until 1923 when white settlers formed the Responsible Government which enjoyed relative independence from Britain.

[59] S. P. Oliver, *Many Treks made Rhodesia*, reprint edition (Bulawayo: Books of Rhodesia, 1975). Rhodes was willing to let the Moodie family take up these lager expanses of land in order to counter Portuguese claims to the region.

[60] Rennie, "Christianity, Colonialism and the Origins of Nationalism," 172.

However, contrary to settlers' claims that they were taking up unoccupied land, the NCs for Chipinge acknowledged the fallacy of such claims. One noted that the farms in Gazaland were all occupied by Africans.[61] Another observed that European settlers chose to peg their farms on the exact spots on which Africans were densely settled.[62] The claims that the land was unoccupied were based on the belief that this part of Gazaland was completely deserted when Gungunyana and his Shangani people moved their capital from the Mossurize valley to Bileni in southern Mozambique. According to Rhodes, the objective of the Moodies' Trek (1893–1898) to Gazaland was "to go and occupy round Gungunyana's old kraals at the headwaters of the Buzi." He claimed that this was "quite unoccupied land" and warned that if the Europeans did not occupy it soon, the Africans would come and fill it up again.[63] Thus, to European settlers, these lands were empty, unproductive, and ripe for exploitation, resulting in the cruel disruption of colonial conquest, displacement, and agrarian intervention.[64] Gungunyana after all did not take all the people with him down to Bileni and some of those who went with him returned after the Portuguese defeated and exiled him.

Colonial land alienation, accompanied by labor demands, also deprived Africans of the ability to modify the environment. As stated earlier, the European settlers who took up lands on the Zimbabwean side of the border were generally of "Boer" origin, Afrikaans-speaking, and undercapitalized. They were the ones who had become "poor whites" in the Orange Free State of South Africa, where a depression and constant division of farms produced small and uneconomic holdings vulnerable to erosion and loss of soil fertility due to overuse. Their undercapitalization meant that they heavily relied on cheap African labor, thereby interfering with African ability to modify the environment. Through a series of legislation such as the Native Passes Ordinance of 1902 and the Private Locations Ordinance of 1908, the BSAC government compelled Africans to work for three months every year on settler farms under labor tenancy. Settlers enforced this system by eviction and physical force, for example, using the *chamboko* (hide whip) to beat their African tenants. This continued into the 1950s,

[61] *Ibid.*, 178.

[62] *Ibid.*

[63] *Ibid.*

[64] Alexander, *The Unsettled Land*, 1. For more in the politics of land and race in Rhodesia, see Palmer, *Land and Racial Domination in Rhodesia*.

with the NC Chipinge reporting that the employment of tenants under labor agreements was still a popular method resorted to by farmers of his district in order to secure a more dependable labor force.[65]

Colonial land-use patterns such as keeping large tracts of land idle encouraged the growth of vegetation which harbored tsetse flies and increased the incidence of trypanosomiasis. In Mozambique, for instance, the Director of Veterinary Services for the Mozambique Company reported in 1915 that trypanosomiasis was becoming more prevalent because, as the land was being continually alienated, the presence of tsetse flies was "now being noticed, whilst in the olden days, when these places were not invaded by settlers, flies were neither seen nor heard of."[66] He also noted in 1918 that considering the rate at which the Company was fighting the tsetse fly, it would take many years "to clean" even the mildly infested parts of Chimoio. The main reason for it is this, he argued, was that the farms or concessions were too big, with only relatively a minute proportion of land cleared for cultivation purposes. To the Director, trypanosomiasis was likely to make its periodic appearance until the Portuguese settlers cleared larger tracts of land and kept their cattle in fenced areas and fed therein.[67] Colonial land-use patterns therefore encouraged the build-up of tsetse fly populations, leading to outbreaks of trypanosomiasis in the border region.

The Mozambique Company also attempted to control the land although its financial situation and inability to attract white settlers led to dependence on African labor as the most important asset. The Company forced Africans to work in its public works department, building roads and railways and in the extractive industries, such as mining and rubber collection. This system of forced labor continued well into the 1960s.[68] While the Portuguese labor code of 1928 abolished forced labor, save for work on government projects, it was merely replaced by intensified

[65] NAZ, S2827/2/2/5: Report of the Native Commissioner, Chipinga, for the year ending 31st December, 1957.

[66] AHM, FCM, Secretaria Geral—Relatórios, Caixa 131, Pasta 2712: Fourth Annual Report of the Veterinary Department, 1915.

[67] AHM, FCM, Secretaria Geral—Relatórios, Caixa 132, Pasta 2733: Relatório da Repartição de Veterinária, 1918.

[68] William Minter, *King Solomon's Mines Revisited: Western interests and the burdened history of Southern Africa* (New York: Basic Books, 1986), 30. For a detailed discussion of forced labor in central Mozambique, see Allina, *Slavery By Any Other Name*.

methods of recruitment and by mandatory crop-growing.[69] Thus although the Mozambique Company compared its territory to "an unknown country inhabited by a few savages," when it received its charter, it soon realized that the African population was its "most valuable asset" and "African participation in the colonial economy would come at the barrel of the gun."[70] The labor recruitment policies the Mozambique Company instituted were akin to predatory raids, with police even seizing young boys and elderly men. In order to make up for shortfalls in labor supply, the Company aimed at increasing recruitment within Manica and recruiting Africans from other districts, such as Moribane, which became an undeclared labor reserve.[71]

In addition to Moribane, the southern district of Mossurize also became a labor reserve. After several Portuguese attempts to settle in Gogoyo in Mossurize failed, it automatically became a labor reserve, where the Portuguese focused more on controlling the people than controlling the land.[72] Here, the Mozambique Company, just like Portugal herself, lacked the financial resources to move beyond extractive "corporate feudalism,"[73] and as a result, by 1906 the Company had resorted to extracting labor and natural resources. It forced villagers in and around Gogoyo to tap indigenous rubber trees and to work on the Company's projects. Those who refused to work found their way to prisons, where they underwent physical punishment, such as the *palmatória*. Mr. Muchuchu of Zangiro, Mozambique, recalled that *palmatória* involved the beating of palms and soles of the feet. When one started bleeding, the officials put salt on the wounds to exacerbate the pain.[74] The fact that the Mozambique Company was not willing to sacrifice the Mafuse rubber plantation to control tsetse fly was a testimony to the importance they placed in this extractive industry.[75]

As villagers were forced to work on colonial projects, households lost their ability to modify the environment and keep trypanosomiasis in check. In African societies of the border region, men were usually the ones who cleared land for agriculture by cutting down vegetation and burning it,

[69] M. D. D. Newitt, *A history of Mozambique*, 150.
[70] Allina-Pisano, "Negotiating Colonialism," 3.
[71] Allina, *Slavery By Any Other Name*, 140.
[72] Hughes, *From Enslavement to Environmentalism*, 21.
[73] *Ibid.*, 30.
[74] Interview with Mr. Muchuchu, Zangiro, Mozambique, September 23, 2006.
[75] Swynnerton, "Examination of the tsetse fly problem in North Mossurise," 372.

whereas women were primarily responsible for planting crops, weeding, and household work, with boys being responsible for milking and herding of cattle, goats, and sheep.[76] Thus, women could not readily take over the duties of absent males. This led to the reduction in the size of cultivated land as the women concentrated on lands already cleared, rather than clearing new lands. The absence of men also meant less labor on the fields, leading to further reduction in cultivated lands. Hence, as the cultivated area shrunk, bush encroached, extending the habitat of the tsetse fly.

Prevalence and Control of Trypanosomiasis Under Colonial Rule

As mentioned earlier, colonial conquest, land use, and contradictions in colonial economies led to epidemics of trypanosomiasis throughout colonial Africa. In the Belgian Congo, for example, state-administered public health initiatives to control trypanosomiasis included imposition of *cordon sanitaires*, forcible isolation, and treatment with drugs, such as atoxyl. However, imposing *cordon sanitaires* curtailed the mobility of the Congolese at a time when colonial demands for rubber forced people to be highly mobile. Thus Belgian colonial officials later resorted to sleeping sickness treatment (medical intervention) rather than prevention by use *cordon sanitaires*.[77] This brings out the clear connection between colonial medical institutions and economic interests.[78] British sleeping sickness policies in the Lake Victoria region of East Africa between 1900 and 1950 also provide an important example of the intrusiveness of colonial public health policy. In this region, sleeping sickness control policies involved compulsory massive relocations and intrusive vegetation clearing campaigns which paralleled military campaigns in Europe.[79] These intrusive measures often connected to economic interests which influenced colonial

[76] W. S. Taberer, "Mashonaland Natives," *Journal of the Royal African Society* 4, no. 15 (1905): 312.

[77] Lyons, *The Colonial Disease*.

[78] For more on this subject, see Randall M. Packard, *White plague, Black Labor: Tuberculosis and the Political Economy of Health and Disease in South Africa* (Berkeley: University of California Press, 1989).

[79] Kirk Aden Hoppe, "Lords of the Flies: British Sleeping Sickness Policies as Environmental Engineering in the Lake Victoria Region, 1900–1950," Working Papers in African Studies, No. 203, African Studies Center, Boston University, 1995. See also Bell, *Frontiers of Medicine*.

public health in the Belgian Congo and the Lake Victoria region were also implemented in the border area of Mozambique and Zimbabwe.

As the trypanosomiasis situation worsened, colonial officials in Zimbabwe and Portuguese authorities experimented with various control methods, resulting in large-scale destruction of wildlife and vegetation. Tsetse and trypanosomiasis control methods also involved restrictions of movement across the border, de-flying chambers, and the use of residual insecticides. Yet, while these tsetse fly and trypanosomiasis control measures were constant and pervasive, they were ineffective.

The control method employed, whether destruction of game or vegetation clearing, was determined by the species of tsetse flies and their ecology. For *G. morsitans* which was largely dependent on large game, officials attempted to control trypanosomiasis by killing wild animals. This was followed by African settlement whenever possible. *G. morsitans* was by far the most important vector of trypanosomiasis in Mozambique, covering three quarters of the colony. However, for the two other species, *G. pallidipes* and *G. brevipalpis*, dependent on certain types of dense forest, officials used vegetation clearings on the border region. These two species fed on small game animals. This meant that the method of game destruction could not practically be applied to the control of these two species of tsetse. Hence, officials applied vegetation clearing as a control measure.

Colonial officials implemented vegetation clearings in different ways. The first method involved "selective clearing" (of upper and lower vegetation elements), which had proved to be the cheapest methods of tsetse control in some East African territories. This form of vegetation control had an added advantage in that it did not cause the decimation or extinction of endemic flora and fauna, nor did it spread the fly. However, colonial authorities in Zimbabwe took no interest in this method and actually dismissed it saying, while selective clearing might eradicate *G. morsitans*, it needed further study and experimentation before it could be safely adopted as an anti-tsetse measure.[80]

What became the favorite method of vegetation control in colonial Zimbabwe and Mozambique, therefore, was the second method which involved barrier clearings along the border, ostensibly to prevent the spread of tsetse flies from Mozambique. The barrier clearing program, known by the locals along both sides of the border as *Machichimana*, did

[80] NAZ, F122/FH/30/1/1: O. J. Sidney, "Tsetse fly control and game eradication," September, 1959.

not have the advantages of the first method. It involved wholesale destruction of indigenous vegetation wherever it was applied, leading to the decimation of endemic flora and fauna.

Outbreaks of trypanosomiasis in Mozambique worried officials in Zimbabwe, who claimed that trypanosomiasis was endemic there. These officials were concerned about the spread of the disease into Zimbabwe. The Mossurize district, for example, experienced severe outbreaks of trypanosomiasis starting in 1915 which triggered an investigation by C. F. M. Swynnerton in 1918. Swynnerton discovered that although Mzila's measures had driven the fly from a large piece of deciduously wooded country, the fly never abandoned its permanent haunts except on the Save and in the cleared portions of Gogoyo area and the Mwangezi. Thus within eight years after Mzila relaxed the measures in 1889, the fly began re-occupying its old haunts and new areas.[81] This was a result of the increase in the deciduous wooding close to the border and an explosion of wildlife due to a reduction in human population after Gungunyana took some people to Bileni. "Up to a very few years ago cattle were still kept successfully in Mossurise within a few miles of the British border from Puizisi [Pwizizi] to Maruma, and from Spungabera to Inyamgamba," wrote Swynnerton, but these "except the Spungabera cattle, which have suffered, have been largely wiped out by successive attacks of nagana [trypanosomiasis], especially during the last three years."[82]

Of great concern to Colonial Zimbabwean officials was that the trypanosomiasis outbreaks in Mozambique coincided with isolated cases in the border areas of Zimbabwe. After the District Veterinary Surgeon (hereafter DVS) for Chipinge district reported the presence of trypanosomiasis at Springvale farm, in 1915 Zimbabwe's Chief Veterinary Surgeon (hereafter CVS) investigated outbreaks of animal trypanosomiasis on Tarka, Springvale, East Leigh, and Mt. Selinda farms along the eastern border. While he concluded that there had been few deaths and did not detect any tsetse flies on these farms, he still hinted that tsetse flies were known to be plentiful a few miles across the border.[83] The CVS claimed that buffalo and big game frequently crossed the border into the grazing grounds of all the cattle concerned. He was not surprised at all that these

[81] Swynnerton, "Examination of the tsetse fly problem in North Mossurise," 372.

[82] *Ibid.*

[83] NAZ, V1/10/6: Trypanosomiasis—Melsetter District, letter from the Chief Veterinary Surgeon to the Director of Agriculture, Southern Rhodesia, 28th July, 1915.

cattle got fly struck because he thought they had come into contact with cattle which had been moved from the low *veldt* (low lying areas) in Portuguese Territory and his evidence for this was the presence of "some very cheap cattle in the district" along the border since 1914.[84]

In order to control the spread of tsetse in this border area, Colonial Zimbabwean officials began to implement barrier clearings in 1918, although they soon abandoned them because of the influenza pandemic. However, Colonial Zimbabwean officials were still concerned about the deteriorating situation in Portuguese East Africa, where the director of veterinary services in the Mozambique Company reported trypanosomiasis-related cattle deaths in several areas in 1918, including Mossurize, Siluvu Hills, Villa Machado, Muda, and Budzi.[85]

As a result of the perceived potential of tsetse flies to spread to Zimbabwe from Mozambique, in 1920 the CVS assured European farmers that should there be any indication of the movement of game inward from Portuguese Territory, officials in Zimbabwe were prepared to allow the shooting of game in a defined belt.[86] Yet, while European settlers in Zimbabwe rushed to blame trypanosomiasis on Mozambique, there were other explanations for these cases of trypanosomiasis other than diffusion from Mozambique. Environmental factors, for instance, were central to the distribution of tsetse and trypanosomiasis as demonstrated earlier in this chapter. As the CVS noted, these cases could have been a result of tsetse fly having extended the usual habitats as a result of the heavy rains in the previous season.[87] He thought the tsetse fly could have established themselves in small enclaves on some farms but would recede with a return of normal seasons. The idle land on settler farms in the border region also contributed to this temporary build-up of tsetse flies. The question of idle land in Zimbabwe emerged after 1900 as the colonial administration

[84] NAZ, V1/10/6: Trypanosomiasis—Melsetter District, letter from the District Veterinary Surgeon, Melsetter District, to the Government Veterinary Surgeon, 20 July, 1915.

[85] AHM, FCM, Secretaia Geral, Relatórios Caixa 132, Pasta 2733: Relatório da Repartição de Veterinária, 1918.

[86] NAZ, V1/10/6: Trypanosomiasis—Melsetter District, letter from the District Veterinary Surgeon, Southern Rhodesia, to the Secretary, Eastern Border Farmers' Association, Chipinga, 11th February, 1920. The CVS was responding to a request from the Eastern Border Farmers' Association that certain measures be taken to prevent tsetse flies from getting established in the Melsetter district.

[87] NAZ, V1/10/6: Trypanosomiasis—Melsetter District, letter from the Chief Veterinary Surgeon to the Director of Agriculture, Southern Rhodesia, 28th July, 1915.

attempted to reverse the results of reckless land alienation in the 1890s by enforcing "beneficial occupation" as a condition to title and ownership. However, the resident magistrate in Chipinge district defended the Boer farmers, arguing that they had demonstrated "beneficial occupation" and that it was the colonial administration's fault to make grants to people without means.[88] This idle land, usually wooded, then provided temporary habitats for tsetse fly during the rainy season.

By 1922, Portuguese veterinarians appeared to be giving up all hope of raising cattle in Mossurise district in the southern portion of the border region. As the Department of Veterinary Services claimed in 1922, there were only a few African-owned cattle in this district. To him, this meant it was "scarcely worthwhile" to consider this district as a cattle-raising area because of great distances from possible markets and the impossibility of bringing cattle safely through the fly-belts.[89]

Fearing the spread of *G. morsitans* from Mozambique, colonial officials in Zimbabwe commenced "controlled discriminate game destruction" in the border region in 1925.[90] By this method, officials argued, the larger game animals on which *G. morsitans* alone could thrive would be reduced in numbers enough to kill the tsetse flies by starvation in a belt (usually about 20 miles wide) along the boundary of infestation.[91]

However, these trypanosomiasis control efforts targeting wild animals only achieved limited success. In 1929, the Colonial Zimbabwean Director of Veterinary Research lamented, for "several years large sums of money have been spent in the endeavour to eliminate the 'fly' by eradicating the game upon which it is thought to be dependent, but these operations have not proved entirely successful."[92] Officials therefore resorted to discriminatory practices in the provision of veterinary services. The Director of Veterinary Research made this clear when he said, "In the meantime, efforts have been made by my Department to deal with the problem from

[88] Rennie, "Christianity, Colonialism and the Origins of Nationalism," 175.

[89] AHM, FCM, Secretaia Geral, Relatórios Caixa 132, Pasta 2742: Relatório da Repartição de Veterinária, 1922.

[90] NAZ, S483/53/2 Trypanosomiasis and Tsetse fly, 1948–1950: Coleman, Secretary to the Prime Minister, to the Chief Secretary, Central African Council, Salisbury, 14th April, 1950.

[91] *Ibid.*

[92] Southern Rhodesia: Report of the Director of Veterinary Research for the Year 1928, presented to the Legislative Assembly in 1929, 5.

another angle, namely, by endeavouring to save the lives of animals belonging to [European] settlers who have ventured into fly-infested areas."[93]

Confronted by a worsening trypanosomiasis situation, colonial officials in Zimbabwe renewed efforts to use barrier clearings in 1932, with the clearing of a 40-mile front of the border in the Chipinge district.[94] The width of this clearing was between one and three miles. It was maintained by slashing back regrowth and by the "judicious use of fire." In fact, a Colonial Zimbabwean Committee of Inquiry reported that the "judicious use of fire" was "a valuable secondary weapon in the hands of the tsetse reclamation officer."[95] Veterinary officers therefore extensively used fire in Chipinge district to compliment barrier clearing. Without vegetation clearing, the use of fire would have been less effective as the Colonial Zimbabwean Chief Entomologist noted that the tsetse fly areas in Zimbabwe consisted largely of either *Mopane* forest (where grass was usually thin and scanty, or sometimes completely absent), or poorly grassed *Mufuti (Brachystegia woodiana)* forest.[96] The total area cleared was approximately 60,000 acres and was replaced with grass.

Although Colonial Zimbabwean officials argued that tsetse flies seldom, if ever, crossed the barrier clearing, tsetse flies, in fact, crossed the clearing during periods of heavy rainfall. As a result, *G. morsitans* covered the entire eastern bank of the Save River by 1933. In the areas around Mt. Selinda and Chipinge, officials claimed that *G. pallidipes* and *G. brevipalpis* were encroaching from their haunts in Mozambique. Thus in 1934 trypanosomiasis control officials extended the border clearing southward from the Chiredza valley past Mt. Selinda to the southernmost beacon of Jersey. This was done in an attempt to protect Gungunyana, Mt. Selinda, Jersey, and other farms along this border area.[97] Officials attributed the occurrence of a few cases behind the clearing to either the ineffectiveness

[93] Southern Rhodesia: Report of the Director of Veterinary Research for the Year 1928, presented to the Legislative Assembly in 1929, 5.

[94] NAZ, F122/FH/30/1/1; O. J. Sidney, "Tsetse fly control and game eradication," September, 1959.

[95] Committee of Inquiry on Tsetse and Trypanosomiasis in Southern Rhodesia, Federation of Rhodesia and Nyasaland (Salisbury: Government Printer, 1954), 8.

[96] R.W. Jack, "The Tsetse fly problem in Southern Rhodesia," Reprinted from *Rhodesia Agricultural Journal*, Bulletin No. 892, May 1933, 14.

[97] Report of the Secretary, Department of Agriculture and Lands for the year 1934, Southern Rhodesia, 19. Gungunyana was an area named after the grandson of Soshangane.

of the clearing itself or a few flies having been present in Zimbabwe and then cut off by the clearing.

Border clearing continued through 1937, with the NC Chipinge reporting that a "gang of Natives" was employed under European supervision in clearing trees and bush from a strip of land along the eastern border, with the objective of checking the advance of tsetse flies.[98] Yet even this aggressive effort at vegetation clearing did not succeed in checking the advance of the fly. In 1939, following the heavy rains of 1938, Colonial Zimbabwean veterinarians claimed that tsetse flies had advanced from Mozambique into the Chipinge sub-district (Chimanimani), causing settler farmers "much loss and concern."[99]

In the meantime, it appeared that the tsetse problem on the Portuguese side got worse. As a result, in September 1941, officials from Zimbabwe and South Africa requested permission to enter Portuguese East Africa, which the Portuguese granted, to study the "spread of Morsitans."[100] These officials were Dr. P. J. du Toit, the Director of Veterinary Services of South Africa, with his two associates, and two officials from Zimbabwe, Mr. B.A. Mayhill, the CVS, as well as two entomologists, Mr. K. W. Jack and Mr. J. K. Chorley.

Due to the gravity of the matter, Portuguese authorities cooperated with their counterparts in Zimbabwe on the control of trypanosomiasis. According to colonial officials in Zimbabwe, the Portuguese government, in response to overtures made by the government of Southern Rhodesia, had generously declared a large area in Portuguese East Africa along the border, east of Melsetter district, an open area for the destruction of all classes of game.[101] Although they were doubtful whether much relief would be obtained along that portion of the border infested with the tsetse flies *G. brevipalpis* and *G. pallidipes*, that is, the section running from the Pwizizi River, south, to the Musirizwi River, they still believed that

[98] NAZ, S1563: Report of the Native Commissioner, Chipinge, for the year ending 31st December, 1937.

[99] Report of the Secretary, Department of Agriculture and Lands for the year 1939, Southern Rhodesia, 5. These cases occurred in the Rusitu valley, leading to a number of deaths among African-owned cattle in the Ngorima reserve and adjoining Native Purchase Area. See NAZ, S235/517: Report of the Assistant Native Commissioner, Melsetter, for the year ended 31st December, 1939.

[100] *Ibid*.

[101] J. K. Chorely, "Tsetse Fly Operations: Short Survey of the Operations by Districts for the Year ending December, 1943," *The Rhodesia Agricultural Journal* 41, no. 1 (1944): 413.

because *G. morsitans* occurred on the Budzi River, the harassing of the big game close to the border could help in controlling the tsetse flies.

However, colonial officials in Zimbabwe doubted the efficacy of game destruction to control *G. brevipalpis* and *G. pallidipes*, because these species of tsetse were more dependent on the presence of vegetation and small game than the big game (buffaloes and elephants) that Portuguese officials were targeting. *G. brevipalpis* and *G. pallidipes* were not "game tsetse fly." The destruction of wild animals in this area followed consultations made in 1939, when Dr. Carlos Ramos, the Director of Veterinary Services in the Mozambique Company government, asked for rifles and ammunition to use for hunting wild animals along the border. In response to this request, J. K. Chorley, then Chief Entomologist of Rhodesia, indicated that his government had agreed to loan the Mozambique Company 20 Martini-Henry rifles and to sell 3000 rounds of ammunition, a consignment delivered to the Veterinary Department of the Mozambique Company at Macequece.[102]

In their control efforts, the Portuguese authorities employed 20 licensed African hunters to kill wild animals along the border. They hunted along the valleys of the Rusitu, Buzi, Mossurize, and Save Rivers. The preferred animals were buffaloes and elephants despite Swynnerton's findings. Swynnerton had warned categorically in 1921 that any attempt in northwest Mossurise to "destroy the fly by starving it in its permanent haunts is doomed to failure if the bush-pigs, and perhaps the baboons also, are not destroyed; and the destruction of the pigs in this type of country is not easy."[103] Yet in January 1942, the *Chefe* of the district of Mossurize indicated that he had deployed 20 hunters to hunt the buffaloes and elephants.[104]

As proof of the ineffectiveness of colonial trypanosomiasis control programs, veterinarians in Zimbabwe reported in 1942,

> Unhappily, the long threatened extension of tsetse fly from Portuguese East Africa into the southern portion of the Melsetter district has now assumed very serious dimensions. It is evident that border clearings of forest and

[102] AHM, FCM, Negoçios Indigenas Processos—Assistencia Social, Culturas Indigenas, 1931–42, Caixa 7, pasta 34.

[103] Swynnerton, "Examination of the tsetse problem in North Mossurise," 337.

[104] AHM, FCM, Negoçios Indigenas Processos, 1931–42, Caixa 7, pasta 34: "Caça ás espécies selvagens," *Chefe* of Mossurise District, to the Governor of the Territory of Manica and Sofala, 2 January, 1942.

> bush, as a greater protection against the incursion of *G. pallidipes* and *G. brevipalpis* must immediately be widened and extended southwards, whilst other measures must be adopted to combat the approach of *G. morsitans*, now located in considerable density within six miles of the international boundary. The threat to stock farming in the South Melsetter district is grave and should [the] fly become permanently established there in numbers, the risk of its spread to our south-eastern ranching areas cannot be ignored.[105]

The year 1942 was also when the Mozambique Company ended its operations in Mozambique. The transition from Company administration to the colonial administration and the Second World War demands contributed to the relaxation of tsetse and trypanosomiasis control measures, which included border supervision. In 1945 the area below Chikore recorded heavy losses of cattle to trypanosomiasis all along the border on a front of about 60 miles.[106] A year later, the NC Chipinge reported that a strip along the Anglo-Portuguese border south of beacon 104 was infested with tsetse fly and that African-owned cattle were suffering from trypanosomiasis. He said that African hunters were employed there on the destruction of game, but their efforts were not effective as the flies had encroached farther into the colony in the area where the hunters were operating.[107]

However, even with these dismal assessments of game destruction, colonial officials in Zimbabwe still enforced game destruction as the principal control measure against *G. morsitans*, leading to widespread decimation of wildlife.[108] Tsetse and trypanosomiasis control led to the killing of 24,351 wild animals in 1946, 16,802 in 1947, and 22,160 in 1948,

[105] Report of the Secretary, Department of Agriculture and Lands for the year 1942, Southern Rhodesia, 10.

[106] Report of the Secretary, Department of Agriculture and Lands for the year 1945, Southern Rhodesia, 65.

[107] NAZ, S1051: Report of the NC Chipinge, for the year ended 31st December, 1946.

[108] The animals killed included the elephant, hippopotamus, rhinoceros, zebra, giraffe, buffalo, wildebeest, eland, roan, sable, kudu, hartebeest, sassaby, waterbuck, nyala, bushbuck, impala, oribi, steinbok, duikerbok, duiker, suni, sundry small antelopes, warthog, bushpig, baboon, monkey, lion, leopard, hyena, jackal and other carnivores, small rodents and other mammals, gemsbok, reedbuck, klipspringer, cheetah, wild cat, lynx, antbear, and some unclassified animals.

colony-wide.[109] By 1952, trypanosomiasis control measures had resulted in the killing of 486,206 wild animals and this number rose to 666,009 by January 31, 1959.[110] Thus wild animals were "mercilessly slaughtered" in order to establish buffer zones between trypanosomiasis resistant game (disease carriers) and European-owned land or farms.[111] Hence, much of the pressure to eliminate game came from white farmers and missionaries on the edges of the tsetse fly belt who demanded a clear policy to protect them and their livestock from an epidemic similar to that in the lake region of Uganda between 1898 and 1905 when one-quarter of the entire human population died of from trypanosomiasis.[112]

On the Portuguese side the Missão de Combate às Tripanossomiases (Mission to Combat Trypanosomiases) was also involved in game destruction in combination with other measures. Between 1947 and 1956, the Missão de Combate às Tripanossomiases killed as many as 71,475 wild animals.[113] Although officials claimed that the number of mammals destroyed each year was only a small proportion of the existing game, there was no way of knowing how many game animals were present in any given area.[114]

As a result of this "merciless slaughter" of fauna, by the 1950s, only small herds of elephants, mostly calves could be seen emerging from the forest of Mossurize "near the frontier, in search of scrub and other plants that grow in the saltish lands of the littoral."[115] This was part of the seasonal migration of elephants in the region.

Yet even with this wholesale destruction of these elephants, there was no relief to the trypanosomiasis situation. The NC Chipinge reported in 1955 that trypanosomiasis spread from Muumbe, Mwangezi, Gwenzi, Ndima, and Chisumbanje dipping tank areas to six new dipping areas of

[109] J. A. Wheelan, "A Review of the Tsetse fly situation in S. Rhodesia, 1948," *Rhodesia Agricultural Journal* 46, no. 4 (1949): 319.

[110] NAZ, F122/FH/30/1/1: O. J. Sidney, "Tsetse fly control and game eradication," September, 1959.

[111] Roben Mutwira, "Southern Rhodesian Wildlife Policy (1890–1953): A Question of Condoning Game Slaughter?" *Journal of Southern African Studies* 15, no. 2 (1989): 250.

[112] *Ibid.*, 257.

[113] NAZ, F122/FH/30/1/1: O. J. Sidney, "Tsetse fly control and game eradication," September, 1959.

[114] *Ibid.*

[115] Mozambique, Commissão de Caça, *Hunting in Mozambique*, A monograph presented by the Mozambique Hunting Committee on the Occasion of the African Tourism 4th Congress held in September 1952 at Lourenço Marques, 42–43.

Chibunji, Chibuwe, Gumira, Dakate, Emerald, and Kondo, resulting in heavy mortality.[116] He also said that while the clearing of bush on the Anglo-Portuguese border continued throughout the year, considerable sections of the approximate 20 miles of fencing on the 55 mile stretch from the Rusitu River to the international beacon 96 were in poor repair, "possibly due to clandestine movement of stock and natives."[117] The problem with the border was that it cut across common grazing grounds, disrupting seasonal movements of cattle, particularly in years of drought, and 1954 had witnessed a drought that reduced pastures for domestic animals. It also limited the mobility of Africans, who had to carry passes and seek permission whenever they wanted to travel outside the areas designated for them. The American Board missionary at Mt. Selinda, Dr. Thompson, for instance, was perturbed by the Portuguese directive that Africans make a three-day trip to Spungabera to secure permission to visit a relative who might live just across the border.[118]

Due to the worsening trypanosomiasis situation, colonial officials in Zimbabwe commenced selective clearing of the southern-most portion of the Save Division, the area to the east of the confluence of the Mkwasini and Save Rivers, by clearing along the Anglo-Portuguese border through the Mossurize valley with the cooperation of Portuguese authorities. These efforts, geared toward tsetse control, were complemented by game destruction. For instance, in 1956 the NC Chipinge reported that an entomologist had, for six months, been involved in the destruction of game in the Save tsetse fly control area. The hunters involved received 22 shillings and 6 pence per year after the colonial government banned the sale of meat and hides as a form of payment.[119] In addition, these officials made representations to the Portuguese Commandant at Spungabera to stop all donkey traffic across the border, but in spite of these precautions and the

[116] NAZ, S2817/2/2/3: Report of the Native Commissioner, Chipinga, for the year ending 31st December, 1955. All in all about 1425 cattle were lost to trypanosomiasis. The first five dipping tank areas had been infected since 1952.

[117] NAZ, S2827/2/2/3: Report of the Native Commissioner, Chipinga, for the year ending 31st December, 1955.

[118] Rennie, "Christianity, Colonialism and the Origins of Nationalism," 320.

[119] NAZ, S282/2/2/4: Report of the NC Chipinge, for the year ended 31st December, 1956.

construction of an eight-mile eight-strand barbed wire fence, tsetse flies continued to be a problem.[120]

As wholesale vegetation clearing decimated endemic flora, colonial officials in Zimbabwe replaced it with fast-growing exotic species such as eucalyptus, wattle, and pine trees for commercial purposes. The Forest Commission led these reforestation efforts that included planting blocks of eucalyptus on the Zona Tea Estate (originally part of Mt. Selinda Farm, belonging to the American Board Mission).[121] Although these officials argued that exotic plantations could not provide permanent tsetse fly habitats,[122] these plantations contributed to the existence of temporary foci of infection, particularly during the wet season, worsening the tsetse fly situation in the border region. The director of Tsetse and Trypanosomiasis Control and Reclamations, for instance, reported in 1958 that the increase in tree plantations among tea estates was complicating the maintenance of the border defense scheme.[123] These exotic species were also detrimental to the environment because they siphoned all the nutrients from the soil leading to loss of fertility. Fertile fields became barren after eucalyptus trees were planted.

However, despite sacrificing endemic flora, trypanosomiasis problems continued. In his report for 1958, J. Ford, then Director of Tsetse and Trypanosomiasis Control and Reclamation in Zimbabwe, indicated just how serious the trypanosomiasis situation had become. He said that the task of re-organizing his Department to adopt techniques of tsetse control

[120] NAZ, S2827/2/2/5: Report of the Native Commissioner, Chipinga, for the year ending 31st December, 1957. Commandants were Portuguese officials responsible for the administration and governance of districts and sub-districts of the Mozambique Company's Territory of Manica and Sofala. They served under the governor of the territory at Beira and their duties involved the exercise of minor judicial powers, the collection of "native" and other taxes, issuing licenses, opening and maintaining roads, and conducting the annual census. According to R. C. F. Maugham, the Commandant "is judge, magistrate, conveyancing barrister, chief of public works, receiver of taxes, supervisor and collector of revenues, chief of police, postmaster, and keeper of Government stores; he is the advisor of all, the friend of the native, the father of his district." For more on this, see R. C. F. Maugham, Portuguese East Africa: The History, Scenery, and Great Game of Manica and Sofala (London: John Murray, 1906), 31–35. Maugham was the H. B. M. Consul for the Districts of Mozambique and Zambezia, and for the Territory of Manica and Sofala.

[121] NAZ, F122/400/7/35/3: Minutes of a meeting of the Tsetse and Trypanosomiasis Control Committee, 6th March, 1958.

[122] *Ibid.*

[123] NAZ, F122/FH/30/1/1: Report of the Director of Tsetse and Trypanosomiasis Control and Reclamation for the year ended 30th September, 1958.

other than game destruction was hampered by a general deterioration of the trypanosomiasis situation in the eastern and southeastern parts of Zimbabwe.[124] He noted that during the summer months the infection rate among cattle on the eastern border farms increased to a peak higher than in any year since 1943 when officials diagnosed 270 infections. When tsetse control officials surveyed the area south of the Lundi River after the rains had ceased, they concluded that extensive advances of tsetse fly, both *G. morsitans* and *G. pallidipes* had occurred since 1956 in a southerly and westerly direction.

Officials attributed this increase in trypanosomiasis incidence to heavy rainfall during the mid-1950s. "It appears that during the wet season," Entomologist R. J. Phelps observed in 1958, "tsetse invaded Southern Rhodesia via the Nyamadzi and Busi river systems."[125] However, these cases also demonstrated the ineffectiveness of control methods as officials asserted that these tsetse flies crossed the clearing which was at least one mile wide. Phelps therefore suggested treating a narrow strip of forest across the full width of these river valleys, both on the eastern and western edges of the clearing with a residual insecticide to prevent future invasions of tsetse.

Ford later realized, however, that the tsetse problem was an ecological one, which impinged upon many fields of rural activity.[126] Ford therefore set up a system of "local Trypanosomiasis Committees" consisting of a Native Commissioner as Chairman, together with a Government Veterinary Officer and a Tsetse Entomologist. The main purpose of these committees was to coordinate tsetse and trypanosomiasis control. According to Ford,

> The tsetse programme and the prophylactic and therapeutic measures carried out by the Veterinary Department can be outlined and explained to representatives of other departments as well as the local farming community and the need for collaboration in such matters as control of cattle movement, grass fires, etc., explained. On the other hand, developmental schemes of various kinds, e.g. native settlement schemes, road building, labour

[124] NAZ, F122/FH/30/1/1: Report of the Director of Tsetse and Trypanosomiasis Control and Reclamation for the Year Ended 30th September, 1958.

[125] NAZ, F122/400/7/35/3: Report on Visit to the Border clearing, 24th April, 1958.

[126] NAZ, F122/FH/30/1/1: Report of the Director of Tsetse and Trypanosomiasis Control and Reclamation for the Year Ended 30th September, 1958.

> recruitment, etc., which may influence or be influenced by anti-tsetse operations, may be discussed.[127]

Ford's suggestion also implies that colonial rule interfered with precolonial trypanosomiasis control methods and casts doubt on the theory of spread of infection from Mozambique as the sole explanation for Colonial Zimbabwean trypanosomiasis outbreaks.

Ford realized that a new approach was needed to solve the trypanosomiasis problem, which reached crisis proportions in 1958. At that time, the NC Chipinge claimed that tsetse fly had invaded areas up the Save valley and threatened the Musikavanhu Reserve. By his estimates, the tsetse fly area included the entire Musikavanhu Reserve, the entire Save Division, the Ndima Reserve, and all other Native Purchase Areas, leaving only the Mutema Reserve free.

Other tsetse fly and trypanosomiasis control measures involved the restrictions of movement and monitoring of entry points and aerial spraying of chemicals, such as DDT. Under the Rhodesia Tsetse Fly Act (1929), for instance, the Governor had powers to control the movement of stock, motor vehicles, cyclists, and pedestrians from or into proclaimed tsetse fly areas.[128] The Governor could declare any defined area to be a tsetse fly area and make regulations for prohibiting the movement of persons, domestic animals, and vehicles to, from, or within fly areas, restricting such movement to certain defined routes and to fixed periods of the day or night. The Act also made provisions for the inspection of domestic animals and vehicles. These inspections were geared toward the detection and removal of tsetse from people, animals, and vehicles. Contravention of these regulations was an offence punishable by a fine not exceeding $10 or, in the case of default of payment, to imprisonment not exceeding one month.[129]

Owing to the fact that tsetse control officials argued that tsetse flies, particularly *G. morsitans, G. swinnertoni*, and *G. pallidipes*, could be carried for long distances on vehicles and shorter distances on cyclists and pedestrians, colonial officials in Zimbabwe established gates on the eastern border to inspect cars, cyclists, and pedestrians. The NC Chipinge, for

[127] *Ibid.*

[128] Committee of Inquiry on Tsetse and Trypanosomiasis, 9.

[129] Maria-Theresa Tarutira, "A Review of Tsetse and Trypanosomiasis in Southern Rhodesia: Economic significance up to 1955," M. A. Thesis, Department of History, University of Zimbabwe, March 1988, 40.

instance, claimed that motor transport was responsible for spreading the fly in certain cases and that "natives travelling on foot through fly belts introduce[d] them among cattle."[130] The inspections involved the use of de-flying chambers which served two purposes, to prevent the transportation of tsetse into fly-free areas and to provide an index of the density of tsetse fly in the areas through which traffic had traveled. Officials at the Mt. Selinda border gate sometimes caught tsetse flies in cars from Mozambique.[131] While this shows that there was some spread of tsetse flies between the colonies, it also affirms the degree of harassment that pedestrians endured on the border. In the mid-1970s, officials began spraying DDT on a barrier strip along the eastern border.

African Reaction

Colonial officials feared that movement across the border would pose serious threats to public health and so sought to restrict the mobility of cattle keepers. As a result, in some cases, Africans who crossed the border into Mozambique had their cattle immediately seized and destroyed by veterinary officials and the border police.[132] While these officials emphasized the importance of supervising the border, not much thought was given to seasonal movements of cattle. The border affected cattle keepers and it was not surprising that cattle keepers sometimes broke border cattle and game fences as a way of resisting these measures, but also because they had no other alternative without adequate pasture for their livestock.

Resistance to trypanosomiasis control measures took many forms. In Mozambique authorities reported in 1941 that in the district of Mossurize, African-owned cattle suffered heavy casualties because the cattle keepers, being "naturally superstitious and rebellious," concealed the major portions of their herds from the authorities.[133] As a result, these cattle perished in large numbers because they were not treated for trypanosomiasis. Similarly, in 1955 officials in Zimbabwe claimed, "local natives will not

[130] NAZ, S1051: Report of the Native Commissioner, Chipinga, for the year ended 31st December, 1946.

[131] NAZ, S3107/1/6: Mount Selinda—Tsetse fly Border Gate: Traffic Control—Eastern Districts, Chipinga—Mount Selinda Border Gate.

[132] See Dube, "'In the Border Regions of the Territory of Rhodesia'"

[133] AHM, FCM, Secretaia Geral, Relatórios Caixa 130, Pasta 2695: Relatório da Repartição de Veterinária, 1941. My translations.

hunt where directed."[134] These officials were concerned because their surveys that same year revealed a heavy build-up of *G. morsitans* in Mozambique from the Ndanga River north of Makoho to the Save-Lundi junction in Zimbabwe. These seemingly irrational behaviors of Africans were prompted by their distrust of colonial trypanosomiasis control methods and the evidence that the measures were ineffective.

African hunters resented game laws imposed by the colonial government, which took away their rights to wildlife. These hunters could not hunt at will when they needed food, but had to hunt animals they could not eat simply to comply with colonial tsetse control demands. To make the best of the need to comply with such demands, Africans resorted to selling game meat and hides, but it was not long before colonial officials clamped down on this activity. In 1956, for example, the Director of Tsetse and Trypanosomiasis Control and Reclamation in Zimbabwe was convinced that the reduction in the area of operations, the concentration of hunters between fences, and the prohibition on the sale of meat and hides would lead to greater control over the activities of hunters and would drastically curtail African traffic into and from tsetse areas and with it the transportation of fly.[135]

Interviews with residents of the border areas show that people still recall trypanosomiasis measures, such as clearings. Mr. Muchuchu of Zangiro, Mozambique, recalled that the greater proportion of border clearings was on the Zimbabwean side of the border to prevent tsetse flies from infecting cattle. He said that Africans knew tsetse bites could cause disease, but argued that it was primarily the sucking of blood by the flies that would result in a shortage of blood in the person or animal affected, causing the disease.[136] He thought that the way Europeans treated the disease in hospitals was to add more blood (blood transfusion) while administering some drugs. This misunderstanding of trypanosomiasis causation and healing might have also contributed to African mistrust of hospitals in the early decades of colonial rule. Africans feared that their blood would be taken in the hospital, that they would be killed, or that another person's blood would be put into their bloodstream. Blood was sacred

[134] NAZ, F122/FH/30/1/1: Annual Report of the Director of Tsetse and Trypanosomiasis Control and Reclamation for the Year Ended 30th September, 1955.

[135] NAZ, F122/400/7/35/2: Annual Report of the Acting Director of Tsetse and Trypanosomiasis Control and Reclamation for the Year Ended 30th September, 1956.

[136] Interview with Mr. Muchuchu, Zangiro, Mozambique, September 23, 2006.

and the mixing of blood was detestable to them. This issue of the significance of blood in African society is discussed in detail in Chap. 8. This interpretation of disease causation, however, demonstrates that colonial trypanosomiasis control policies were poorly received by Africans because they did not include African understandings of disease causation and healing. As a result, Europeans did not gain greater compliance with disease control from African villagers.

According to Mr. Muchuchu, those forced to slash vegetation to create these clearings were bandits (prisoners) or captives.[137] In Mozambique, this could have meant anybody who resisted colonial authority, particularly those who resisted forced labor. On this subject, Mr. Mbekwa, of Mpanyeya, Mozambique, recalled that colonial officials forced villagers to clear the border by cutting trees and clearing the grass so as to control tsetse fly, which they believed to be the major cause of death in animals and human beings, and that "these tsetse control measures included the destruction of many wild animals at a certain place."[138]

There were, however, differing opinions on the purpose of these clearings. Veterinarians in Zimbabwe reported in 1958 that the "clearing was being maintained [probably by both settlers and Africans] more for pasture improvement [than tsetse control] which was not the function of the Tsetse Control Department."[139] Some villagers from the area around Spungabera still have vivid memories of these control programs. For example, Mrs. Chiphoto of Mamuse, Mozambique, remembered, "the *Machichimana* program involved people cutting down trees along the border to prevent people from crossing with their herds unnoticed," adding, "it was also said to be a control measure for tsetse fly but since many people avoided crossing the border with their cattle, for fear that they would be confiscated, the clearing of the border was then to prevent people from crossing unnoticed."[140] To this, Mr. Mubekapi Matoro of Makubvu, Mozambique, concurred, arguing that *Machichimana* was not primarily for controlling tsetse fly but to prevent Africans from crossing the border unnoticed.[141]

[137] *Ibid.*

[138] Interview with Mr. T. Mbekwa, Mpanyeya, Mozambique, 14 December, 2006.

[139] NAZ, F122/400/7/35/3: Meeting of the Tsetse and Trypanosomiasis Control Committee, Department of Tsetse and Trypanosomiasis and Reclamation, Southern Rhodesia, 9th January, 1958.

[140] Interview with Mrs. Chiphoto, Mamuse, Mozambique, 23 February, 2007.

[141] Interview with Mr. Mubekapi Matoro, Makubvu, Mozambique, January 6, 2007.

Africans residing on the Zimbabwean side of the border also had their own interpretations of colonial veterinary and public health policy. One elder, Mr. F. Mangemba of Maengeni Village in Chipinge, said that border clearing was geared toward checking the movement of animals, such as cattle, as well as checking the movement of certain contaminated products, such as fruits.[142] However, despite fencing and shooting operations, seasonal game movement was responsible for spreading tsetse.[143] This often resulted from breaches of cattle and game fences by wild animals, cattle, and cattle keepers who disliked measures that prevented long-established patterns of transhumance.[144]

In 1961 the NC Chipinge reported on African resistance to tsetse fly and trypanosomiasis control measures by cattle owners at Kondo and Chibuwe who refused to make their cattle available for smearing (to diagnose trypanosomiasis). He claimed that the prosecution of 192 African cattle owners eventually broke the resistance.[145] Although these African cattle owners later cooperated with the colonial authorities by having their cattle inoculated, this incident shows that some villagers disliked government-imposed control measures. In other cases, colonial officials prevented Africans from owning cattle due to fear of trypanosomiasis. The same NC Chipinge reported in 1961 that villagers living in Tamandayi Native Purchase Area had "been pressing for [permission to own cattle] for some time."[146]

In the 1970s the war in Mozambique and the war of independence in Zimbabwe interfered with tsetse and trypanosomiasis efforts. The general insecurity in the countryside complicated control efforts. As a result, the incidence of trypanosomiasis increased. One resident of Chitakatira Village in Zimbabwe, for instance, said that there might have been some

[142] Interview with Mr. F. Mangemba, Maengeni Village, Chipinge, Zimbabwe, 14 January, 2007.

[143] NAZ, F122/400/7/35/3: Minutes of a meeting of the Tsetse and Trypanosomiasis Control Committee, 7th August, 1958.

[144] NAZ, S3708/5/1–2: Monthly reports, Department of Tsetse and Trypanosomiasis control, Southern Rhodesia, 1975–6.

[145] NAZ, S2827/2/2/8: Report of the Native Commissioner, Chipinga, for the year ended 31st December, 1961. Advocate Hebert Chitepo was the first African lawyer in Southern Rhodesia.

[146] *Ibid*. Tamandayi is on the eastern border with Mozambique.

outbreaks of human trypanosomiasis and that some of the people who contracted the disease became insane.[147]

Conclusion

As this chapter has demonstrated, the imposition of colonial rule led to the disruption of tsetse fly ecology and made control of trypanosomiasis difficult. Fears of infection, based on erroneous epidemiology of trypanosomiasis, contributed to the efforts to restrict human and animal mobility within and across territorial boundaries. Although some African societies had developed mechanisms for keeping the tsetse flies and trypanosomiasis in check, colonial officials claimed that these were not effective. In any case, the labor and land demands of the colonial economy would not have allowed for Africans to keep their ability to modify the environment and ensure limited but constant contact with tsetse flies, necessary for the build-up of immunity.

Colonial economies demanded that Africans be dispossessed of their lands, be pushed to the marginal areas, some of which were heavily infested with tsetse flies, and that Africans should provide labor for colonial projects. In both Mozambique and Zimbabwe, forced labor was common at the beginning of colonial rule. Although there was more land alienation in Zimbabwe than in Mozambique, Portuguese labor policies were equally disruptive to the environment. Throughout much of Mozambique's colonial period, Portuguese officials forced Africans to provide labor for European farmers and miners, as well as for building roads and bridges and other colonial projects. In other parts of Mozambique, such as Gogoyo, colonial officials forced Africans into tsetse-infested forests to tap wild rubber and to work for Portuguese settlers. Thus, while there was no large-scale land alienation in the Mozambican portion of the border region, colonial labor conscription and other demands reduced the time Africans devoted to cultivation. All these demands meant that Africans no longer had the ability to modify their environments and control trypanosomiasis.

The imposition of colonial rule therefore had deleterious consequences on the epidemiology of African trypanosomiasis. The large tracts of land that settlers seized from the Africans, kept idle by absentee landlordism, or partially cultivated due to lack of resources, soon became overgrown with

[147] Interview, Chitakatira Village, Mutare South, August 1, 2006.

vegetation, which became havens for tsetse flies. Thus, while there could have been some movement of tsetse from Mozambique into Zimbabwe, the existence of these large expanses of idle land, the introduction of exotic tree species in cleared areas, and African inability to modify the environment created some local foci of infection within Zimbabwe itself.

In addition, the border prevented the continuation of the forms of transhumance which had contributed to protecting cattle from trypanosomiasis. The uplands of Zimbabwe had always served as safe areas to move cattle during the wet season when trypanosomiasis incidence increased in the lowlands of Mozambique. Yet, as this chapter has demonstrated, border game and cattle fences prevented movements of cattle in these micro-environments. Tsetse fly and trypanosomiasis control measures therefore led to the disruption of the African way of life. They caused hardship to many Africans. As Africans and their cattle became buffers to protect Europeans and their cattle from trypanosomiasis, they suffered the most from the effects of changing tsetse ecologies at a time when it was impossible to practice local forms of transhumance that protected cattle from trypanosomiasis and provided fresh pastures.

Confronted by a worsening trypanosomiasis situation, colonial officials resorted to wanton destruction of wildlife and vegetation. Even when there were signs that game eradication was not effective, officials still hailed this method, mercilessly slaughtering wild animals and leading the reduction in wildlife populations in order to protect mostly settler cattle and settlers themselves from disease. Although there were no recorded cases of human trypanosomiasis in the border region, its existence in other parts of the two colonies, coupled with erroneous ideas about the epidemiology of the disease, led to the implementation of stringent control measures by colonial officials. Thus, as long as *G. morsitans* existed, officials for a long time believed that they could trigger an epidemic in humans.

Yet, as this chapter has shown, the African response clearly casts doubt on the intentions and motives of colonial control efforts, demonstrating that public health efforts were routinely interpreted in various ways, in this case, unintended, often revealing other kinds of disagreements and conflicts with regard to what colonialism was about. This response reveals suspicion of colonial policies that were discriminatory in nature and backed up with force of various kinds, such as forced labor, forced or restricted movements, destruction of the environment, slaughter of cattle, and border inspections. In this way, the competing knowledge(s) in the region point to a disruption of local ecologies and local ways of life.

References

Alexander, Jocelyn. *The Unsettled Land: State-making and the Politics of Land in Zimbabwe, 1893–2003*. Oxford: James Currey, 2006.

Allina, Eric. *Slavery By Any Other Name: African Life Under Company Rule in Colonial Mozambique*. Charlottesville: University of Virginia Press, 2012.

Allina-Pisano, Eric. "Negotiating Colonialism: Africans, the State, and the Market in Manica District, Mozambique, 1895–c. 1935." PhD Dissertation, Yale University, May 2002.

Bell, Heather. *Frontiers of Medicine in the Anglo-Egyptian Sudan, 1899–1940*. Oxford: Clarendon Press, 1999.

Bigalke, R. D. "The Important Role of Wildlife in the Occurrence of Livestock Diseases in Southern Africa." In *Infectious Diseases of Livestock, with Special Reference to Southern Africa*. Volume I, edited by J. A. W. Coetzer, G. R. Thomson, R. C. Tustin, and N. P. J. Kriek, 154–163. Cape Town: Oxford University Press, 1994.

Chorely, J. K. "Tsetse Fly Operations: Short Survey of the Operations by Districts for the Year ending December, 1943." *The Rhodesia Agricultural Journal* 41, 1 (1944): 413.

Dube, Francis. "'In the Border Regions of the Territory of Rhodesia, There Is the Greatest Scourge...': The Border and East Coast Fever Control in Central Mozambique and Eastern Zimbabwe, 1901–1942." *Journal of Southern African Studies* 41, 2 (2015): 219–235.

Ford, John. *The Role of the Trypanosomiases in African Ecology: A Study of the Tsetse Fly Problem*. Oxford: Clarendon Press, 1971.

Giblin, James. "Trypanosomiasis Control in African History: An Evaded Issue?" *Journal of African History* 31, 1 (1990): 59–80.

Giblin, James. "Integrating the History of Land Use into Epidemiology: Settler Agriculture as the Cause of Disease in Zimbabwe." Working Paper No. 176 presented as part of the History of Land Use in Africa project of the African Studies Center, Boston University, and the Forest History Society, 1994.

Headrick, Daniel R. "Sleeping Sickness Epidemics and Colonial Responses in East and Central Africa, 1900–1940." *PLOS Neglected Tropical Diseases* 8, 4 (2014): 1–8.

Headrick, Rita, ed. *Colonialism, Health and illness in French Equatorial Africa, 1885–1935*. Atlanta: African Studies Association Press, 1994.

Hoppe, Kirk Aden. "Lords of the Fly: Colonial Visions and Revisions of African Sleeping-Sickness Environments on Ugandan Lake Victoria, 1906–61." *Africa* 67, 1 (1997): 86–105.

Hoppe, Kirk Aden. "Lords of the Flies: British Sleeping Sickness Policies as Environmental Engineering in the Lake Victoria Region, 1900–1950."

Working Papers in African Studies, No. 203, African Studies Center, Boston University, 1995.

Hughes, David M. *From Enslavement to Environmentalism: Politics on a Southern African Frontier*. Seattle: University of Washington Press in association with Weaver Press, Harare, 2006.

Jack, R. W. "The Life Economy of a Tsetse Fly." *The Rhodesia Agricultural Journal* 41, 1/2 (1944): 25–38.

Kjekshus, Helge. *Ecology Control and Economic Development in East African History: The Case of Tanganyika 1850–1950*. Heinemann, London, 1977.

Lyons, Maryinez. *The Colonial Disease: A Social History of Sleeping Sickness in Northern Zaire, 1900–1940*. Cambridge: Cambridge University Press, 1992.

Malowany, Maureen. "Unfinished Agendas: Writing the History of Medicine of Sub-Saharan Africa." *African Affairs* 99 (2000): 325–349.

Mavhunga, Clapperton Chakanetsa. *Transient Workspaces: Technologies of Everyday Innovation in Zimbabwe*. Cambridge, MA: MIT Press, 2014.

Minter, William. *King Solomon's Mines Revisited: Western Interests and the Burdened History of Southern Africa*. New York: Basic Books, 1986.

Mozambique, Commissão de Caça. *Hunting in Mozambique*, A Monograph Presented by the Mozambique Hunting Committee on the Occasion of the African Tourism 4th Congress held in September 1952 at Lourenço Marques.

Mutwira, Roben. "Southern Rhodesian Wildlife Policy (1890–1953): A Question of Condoning Game Slaughter?" *Journal of Southern African Studies* 15, 2 (1989): 250–262.

Newitt, Malyn. *A History of Mozambique*. Bloomington: Indiana University Press, 1995.

Oliver, S. P. *Many Treks Made Rhodesia*, reprint edition. Bulawayo: Books of Rhodesia, 1975.

Palmer, Robin. *Land and Racial Domination in Rhodesia*. Berkeley: University of California Press, 1977.

Phelps, R. J. and Lovemore, D. F. "Vectors: Tsetse Flies." in *Infectious Diseases of Livestock, with Special Reference to Southern Africa*. Volume I, edited by J. A. W. Coetzer, et al., 25–51. Cape Town: Oxford University Press, 1994.

Rennie, John Keith. "Christianity, Colonialism and the Origins of Nationalism among the Ndau of Southern Rhodesia, 1890–1935." PhD Thesis, Department of History, Northwestern University, 1973.

Swynnerton, C. F. M. "Examination of the Tsetse Problem in North Mossurise, Portuguese East Africa." *Bulletin of Entomological Research* 11, 4 (1921): 315–385.

Taberer, W. S. "Mashonaland Natives." *Journal of the Royal African Society* 4, 15 (1905): 311–336.

Tarutira, Maria-Theresa. "A Review of Tsetse and Trypanosomiasis in Southern Rhodesia: Economic Significance up to 1955." M. A. Thesis, Department of History, University of Zimbabwe, March 1988.

Turshen, Meredith. *The Political Ecology of Disease in Tanzania*. New Brunswick: Rutgers University Press, 1984.

Worboys, Michael. "The Comparative History of Sleeping Sickness in East and Central Africa, 1900–1914." *History of Science* 32 (1994): 89–98.

CHAPTER 6

Cross-Border movements, Smallpox Epidemics, and Public Health

As colonial officials busily set about consolidating their authority, they were soon confronted by epidemics. These outbreaks of diseases were partly a result of the ecological changes and greatly enhanced African mobility triggered by the establishment of colonial rule. Hence, it is crucial to examine the influence of the border on the implementation of public health policy against smallpox and its impact on the African people of the border region. The border continued to be productive in generating fears of diffusion of smallpox into Zimbabwe from a supposedly poorly governed Mozambique. Smallpox was among the most dreaded diseases within colonial society because it was highly contagious and deadly. Yet the border was also productive in generating desires among Africans to cross it for various reasons, including to seek work and to attend religious ceremonies. The colonial response, however, was the coercion and social control of Africans through biopolitics.

Although smallpox existed in endemic form before the imposition of colonial rule, colonial intrusion and the labor demands of the colonial economy that encouraged extensive migration from the 1890s onward led to smallpox epidemics. This chapter shows how some precolonial Africans had developed their own public health methods to deal with smallpox. Their resistance to colonial public health measures, particularly vaccination and disease surveillance, must therefore be viewed as a rejection of the legitimacy of racist colonial authority, characterized by paternalism and a host of dehumanizing practices.

F. Dube, *Public Health at the Border of Zimbabwe and Mozambique, 1890–1940*, African Histories and Modernities,
https://doi.org/10.1007/978-3-030-47535-2_6

Smallpox or *Variola* major was an acute contagious disease caused by the variola virus. It raised much fear because it was easily spread from an infected person by coughing, talking, or contact with an infected person's bedding or clothing to any contacts who had not acquired immunity to the disease. Hence, the close proximity and crowded conditions of the mushrooming colonial urban centers, as well as mining and farming compounds, favored transmission. The disease incubated without symptoms in an infected person for about 12 days. After this, smallpox manifested itself with a rising fever, a strong headache, blisters in the throat, and a rash that quickly turned into blisters on the skin.[1] It was often fatal, with 20–30 percent mortality within seven to ten days. For those who survived, recovery took five to six weeks, during which time the patient remained infectious. However, those who survived smallpox acquired lifelong immunity to it, albeit not without cost, as several of them were left "grossly scarred by pockmarks, blind and infertile ... [and] such facial disfigurement was enough to cause depression, self-concealment and even suicide."[2]

Smallpox often occurred in devastating epidemic cycles during the colonial period. However, many intervening outbreaks were probably of the less virulent strains of the variola virus, known as *variola minor* or alastrim, whose occurrence was first recognized at the end of the nineteenth century, almost simultaneously in the southern United States and in Southern and Eastern Africa.[3] Nonetheless, the word smallpox itself, whether mild (alastrim, often mistaken for *variola major*) or virulent, struck fear into many European settlers in Zimbabwe and Mozambique, prompting action. In Zimbabwe, for example, no matter what type of smallpox was encountered, all precautions were taken and all contacts were vaccinated.[4] Early in the colonial period, this was conducted in the form of "vaccination campaigns," where rural villagers were rounded up and forcibly inoculated. African laborers in urban areas, mining, and farming compounds were also vaccinated.

These vaccinations were not restricted to Africans in Zimbabwe. Due to the problems posed by the border in smallpox control programs, the Colonial Zimbabwean Government implemented a policy of vaccinating

[1] Howard Phillips, *Epidemics: The Story of South Africa's Five Most Lethal Human Diseases* (Athens, Ohio University Press, 2012), 15–16.

[2] *Ibid.*, 16.

[3] Frank Fenner, "Smallpox: Emergence, Global Spread, and Eradication," *History and Philosophy of the Life Sciences* 15 (1993): 404.

[4] Gelfand, *A Service to the Sick*, 21–22.

all labor recruits at ports of entry, although some migrants still managed to enter Zimbabwe using undesignated ports of entry dotted along the lengthy border between Mozambique and Zimbabwe. This pervasive monitoring of the border and mandatory vaccination at entry points increased illegal immigration, potentially spreading smallpox.

In Zimbabwe, officials argued that smallpox diffusion posed a potential danger to the white population, which the colonial government aimed at protecting.[5] In addition, because of its tendency to deplete populations, smallpox was destructive economically by depriving the colonial government of the much-needed labor force. Hence, the colonial government needed to widen the net on health issues to include Africans.

While there was never an effective remedy for smallpox, people around the world developed two preventive measures against smallpox. These measures included variolation, a potentially lethal method of inoculation involving the deliberate introduction of smallpox (variola) virus to a non-sufferer through pus or scabs in a controlled manner in order to induce immunity and vaccination, which involved the transmission of the non-lethal cowpox virus to achieve the same objective.[6]

There is evidence that some precolonial peoples in Zimbabwe, for example, the Ndebele in western Zimbabwe, had already developed public health measures to deal with smallpox, including variolation, isolation, and quarantine. A case in point occurred in 1893, when Lobengula, king of the Ndebele people in western Zimbabwe, ordered an *impi* (regiment) which he had sent north to the Zambezi not to proceed further than Inyoka on its way back to his capital, Bulawayo, because it had contracted smallpox.[7] Lobengula summoned this *impi* to send him the cattle it had

[5] F. Chasokela, "A History of Smallpox in Southern Rhodesia, 1890–1970," B. A. Honors Dissertation (Department of History, University of Zimbabwe, 1985), 16. As for Mozambique, Gerhard Liesegang has also looked at how smallpox, among other factors, such as famines, plagues, and long periods of warfare affected relations of production and distribution in his paper, "Famines, Epidemics, Plagues and Long Periods of Warfare: their effects in Mozambique, 1700–1975," Paper presented at the Conference on Zimbabwean History: Progress and Development, University of Zimbabwe, August 23–27, 1982.

[6] Variolation was practiced in China, the Middle East, and perhaps parts of Africa before 1550, see Phillips, *Epidemics*, 15. Vaccination was developed by a British physician, Edward Jenner, in the 1790s after observing that milk maids in Britain never contracted smallpox. It was later discovered that they got their immunity against smallpox from their exposure to the less virulent cowpox.

[7] NAZ, AOH-59 Oral History: Smallpox, Interview with Mrs. Maore Raridza Mudzongai-Ngomambi (Born in 1896) at Mumugwi, Bindura District, on 8 August 1979, Interviewer:

captured, but otherwise to stay away. According to one elder, Mrs. Maore Raridza Mudzongai-Ngomambi, Lobengula also ordered that "[i]f anyone has a relation who has the disease, he should take the pus from him and make an incision on himself then smear that pus on himself. Then you would fall ill. ... That was the treatment."[8] Similar reports emerged even in the Zimbabwe-Mozambique border region, to the east of Lobengula's territory, where interviewees recalled that people who suffered from smallpox stayed in secluded places near a forest, where their family and relatives brought them food until they recovered from the disease.

When these indigenous efforts are considered, Europeans appear to have brought few new weapons against smallpox. While they understood the cause and means by which smallpox spread, they still lacked treatment for the disease and brought no new ways of diagnosing the disease.[9] The methods the Europeans did bring, isolation and quarantine, were already practiced by some Africans. However, colonial officials added a new element in the health care equation, surveillance, which became crucial in identifying and reporting cases. But some Africans, being aware of the benefits of their own interventions, became resistant to colonial vaccination campaigns. They viewed these campaigns as less effective and as merely policing strategies that undermined traditional medical and religious practices (see Chap. 8) as well as the right of association and assembly.

Outbreaks, Diffusion, and Vaccination

In Southern Africa, there were three severe smallpox outbreaks in Cape Town, South Africa, in 1713, 1755, and 1767.[10] Farther to the north, in Zimbabwe, after ravaging Ndebele armies in the early 1890s, smallpox, which had become routinely endemic in most of Southern Africa, could

Dawson Munjeri. For further details see: AOH/58 Interview with Ngomambi and S. Glass, *Matebele War*, (London: Longmans, 1968).

[8] NAZ, AOH/58 Oral History: Smallpox, Interview held with Mr. Mbangwa Ngomambi (born c. 1877 d. 1983) on 14 July 1979 at Mumugwi, Bindura District, Interviewer: Dawson Munjeri.

[9] William H. Schneider, "The Long History of Smallpox Eradication: Lessons for Global Health in Africa," in *Global Health in Africa: Historical Perspectives on Disease*, ed. James L. A. Webb, JR. and Tamara Giles-Vernick (Athens: Ohio University Press, 2013), 27. See also Eugenia W. Herbert, "Smallpox Inoculation in Africa," *Journal of African History* 16, 4 (1975): 539–559.

[10] Russel S. Viljoen, "Disease and Society: VOC Cape Town, its People and the Smallpox Epidemics of 1713, 1755, and 1767," *Kleio* XXVII (1995): 22–45.

take epidemic form as a result of extremes of poverty, malnutrition, and social dislocation.[11] However, many Shona people of the Zimbabwe-Mozambique border region believed that epidemics of smallpox increased during the colonial period.[12] Similar trends were observed in Eastern Africa, where smallpox became widespread as a consequence of the great extension of trade and communication between the coast and the interior in the nineteenth century.[13]

In the Zimbabwe-Mozambique border region, a case of smallpox was reported in 1899 from the "Coolie Gardens," Mutare, in an Indian man who had recently arrived from Aden.[14] Colonial officials in Zimbabwe responded by posting a police guard around the man's house because his removal was considered risky. Thereafter, several smallpox outbreaks were recorded between 1900 and 1910, but the disease was especially prevalent in 1903–1904 when 80,000 to 90,000 Africans were vaccinated in Zimbabwe, mostly by members of the Native Department.[15]

Portuguese officials also carried out vaccinations. In 1901 Mozambique Company officials requested tubes of vaccine lymph in order to contain an epidemic in Manica and Chimoio.[16] In his annual report for the year ending 1906, the Company's Health Services director wrote, "we continued the vaccination service with the regularity of the previous years. We do not have any epidemic to combat. It is only for prophylaxis that we vaccinated all the natives who passed through these centers of service—Beira, Macequece and Sena."[17] Portuguese officials enforced compulsory vaccination of Africans in any affected district.

Demonstrating the intrusive nature of control measures, a 1909 outbreak in Mutoko, Zimbabwe, outside the border region, with at least 200 cases and 40 deaths, resulted in the use of the police who were reported to have assisted the medical authorities in their efforts to combat the

[11] Terence Ranger, "Plagues of beasts and men; prophetic responses to epidemic in Eastern and Southern Africa," in Terence Ranger and Paul Slack (eds), *Epidemics and Ideas: Essays in the Historical Perception of Pestilence* (Cambridge: Cambridge University Press, 1992), 244.

[12] Interview, Vheremu, Zimbabwe, 24 December, 2006.

[13] Ranger, "Plagues of beasts and men," 244

[14] The Beira Post, September 27, 1899, 3. "Coolie" is a dated and offensive term given to an unskilled indigenous laborer in some Asian countries.

[15] Gelfand, *A Service to the Sick*, 21.

[16] AHM, FCM, Secretaria Geral: Processos, 1892–1942, Varíola e Influenza, 1903–1938, Caixa 130, Pasta 478.

[17] AHM, FCM, Secretaria Geral: Relatórios, Caixa 127, Pasta 2594, Relatório anual dos Serviços de Saúde da Companhia de Moçambique, 1906. My translation.

disease.[18] In 1910, a "systematic vaccination" campaign resulted in government medical officers vaccinating 34,446 Africans. Then, when limited outbreaks of smallpox occurred in Chipinge, in the border region, public health officials forcibly vaccinated 105,450 Africans.

Even more stringent measures were employed from time to time, for example, during an extensive epidemic which occurred in Rusape district in 1913. This outbreak proved challenging to control as the disease spread rapidly from village to village, resulting in the entire district being placed under strict quarantine for almost six months, with 26,147 people vaccinated. In addition, during an outbreak in Gabaza Reserve in 1919, a hut was built for each sick African, who alone was allowed to occupy it, with a trooper, 2 African policemen, 2 African messengers, and 20 African guards setting up a cordon, after which the police and guards and then all within it were vaccinated, including those living in surrounding villages.[19] Colony-wide, in 1921 a total of 168,003 vaccinations were performed by Native Department officials and police and, subsequent to that, 70,324 people were vaccinated in 1922, followed by 214,453 in 1927, and 265,536 in 1928.[20]

On the Mozambican side, comprehensive public health legislation came with the promulgation of the *Regulamento dos Serviços Sanitários do Território* (Regulations for Health Services of the Territory, hereafter *Regulamento*) in 1918. Article 1 of this *Regulamento* stated that the services of public hygiene and sanitary police were to monitor and study the hygiene and physical life of the population in the interest of public health. The other goals included, among other things, promoting the public health, guarding against the introduction of diseases, prevention and control of infectious diseases, promoting the health of public places and habitations, and any other applications of public hygiene relating to the physical well-being of the population.[21]

In Zimbabwe, all the pre-1924 smallpox outbreaks were dealt with using the Cape Colony Public Health Act of 1886 (South Africa), involving medical supervision (surveillance) of the affected area, isolation of patients, and the systematic vaccination of the local population by the

[18] The Beira Post, August 18, 1909, 2.

[19] *Ibid.*, 20.

[20] Gelfand, *A Service to the Sick*, 21.

[21] AHM, FCM, Secretaria Geral: Processos, 1892–1942, Serviços Sanitários, 1897–1941. Caixa 478, Pasta 1786. Governo do Território de Manica e Sofala: Regulamento dos Serviços Sanitários do Território, 1918.

Native Department.[22] However, the promulgation of the Public Health Act in 1925 enhanced the powers of Colonial Zimbabwean officials in public health matters. Some of the major aims of this Act were "to prevent and guard against the introduction of diseases from outside" and "to promote the public health, and the prevention, limitation or suppression of infectious and contagious diseases within the Colony."[23] For the purposes of this Act, the term "infectious disease" referred to the following diseases: smallpox (and any diseases resembling smallpox); chicken pox; typhus fever; plague; Asiatic cholera; leprosy; anthrax; rabies; trypanosomiasis (sleeping sickness); and all forms of tuberculosis. That smallpox topped the list of these infectious diseases was not a mistake. This reflects the anxiety smallpox epidemics generated among European settlers. Smallpox deaths could exceed 30 percent in a community that was "not at least partly immunized," as demonstrated by the 1670–1672 and 1707 smallpox epidemics which occurred on Iceland, with the 1707 outbreak taking a toll of about a third of the population.[24]

Under the provisions of the 1924 Public Health Act, therefore, enormous powers were conferred on local authorities to deal with a smallpox outbreak. For example, these authorities could enforce a 14-day quarantine of any home or factory and could order the examination of people suspected of having smallpox. They could also hold under surveillance, move, and detain or isolate any person suspected of being infected, as well as destroy the possessions of these suspect people and close schools at which smallpox occurred. Also, officials cordoned off affected villages and placed African guards to prevent anyone from entering or leaving the area. Furthermore, local authorities continued to place the sick in special "huts" erected on sites where the patients could receive care, with contacts with suspicious signs, such as fever, being monitored. Finally, officials could and often did order the rest of the people within the cordon to be vaccinated, together with those of surrounding villages. This systematic vaccination was performed by members of the Native Department or the Police Force.[25]

[22] The Rhodesian government used South African public health legislation before the promulgation of its own laws, which were also modeled on the South African ones.

[23] NAZ, S1173/225-227: Infectious Diseases-Public Health Act, 3–4.

[24] Liesegang, "Famines, Epidemics, Plagues and Long Periods of Warfare," 4.

[25] Gelfand, *A Service to the Sick*, 19.

A point worth noting was that prominent among the main aims of Colonial Zimbabwean and Portuguese public health regulations was preventing the *introduction* of infections from outside the colonies. Hence, the Zimbabwe-Mozambique border took center stage in public health policy. Colonial officials in Zimbabwe often blamed smallpox outbreaks on Mozambican migrants because these officials believed the Mozambican public health system was poorly developed. This reflected general Anglophone prejudice on Lusophone colonies. These officials probably exaggerated the extent of diffusion of disease from neighboring Mozambique to conceal the futility of their own public health system. There were, for instance, many local foci of disease because of African resistance to smallpox vaccination.

Nonetheless, the history of smallpox in Zimbabwe shows that the border posed enormous challenges to the adoption of regional smallpox control programs. The lack of a comprehensive cross-border vaccination program, cross-border movements of people, and resistance from some sections of the African population ensured that smallpox remained a major problem in the border region, even in Zimbabwe, where colonial officials prided themselves in having developed more effective and comprehensive control programs than those of Mozambique. Thus, when colonial officials in Zimbabwe learned of the existence of smallpox at Beira in Mozambique in August 1919, they promptly issued an order prohibiting the entry of Africans from Mozambique by train through the Mutare border post, unless these Africans were in possession of a certificate showing they had not been in contact with a case of smallpox for 21 days.[26] This outbreak had started in July 1919 in Beira and was reported to be on the wane by October 1919, after sickening 14 Europeans, 2 "Asiatics," and 396 Africans, resulting in the deaths of 1 "Asiatic" and 73 Africans.[27]

However, some Africans were determined to bypass the border inspections by using alternative routes. Before this waning of the 1919 outbreak, officials in Zimbabwe discovered that an African migrant from Mozambique who had traveled by train from Mutare to Gweru was suffering from smallpox. They claimed that he "was one of a gang which had evaded the railway restrictions by walking from Portuguese Territory through

[26] NAZ, A3/12/29: Smallpox, 1910–1922, Letter from the Secretary, Department of Administrator, to the Town Clerk, Salisbury, Rhodesia, 16th January, 1920.

[27] "Smallpox Figures: Disease Definitely Disappearing," *The Beira News*, Friday, October 24, 1919, 3.

Penhalonga to Mutare where they entrained."[28] That year, several deaths occurred in the outbreak of August 1919 when the infection, which was believed to have originated in Mozambique, spread from east to west, with most of the 120 cases (16 European and 104 African), occurring in Harare, Mutare, Gweru (Gwelo), Kadoma (Gatooma), Nyanga, Chipinge, Chegutu (Hartley), Charter, Mberengwa (Belingwe), and Masvingo (Fort Victoria), resulting in the death of 4 Europeans and 30 Africans. The following year then witnessed 18 separate outbreaks in several areas, including Nyanga, Harare, Mutare, Gweru, Chipinge, Inyati, Mberengwa, Mvuma (Umvuma), Gwanda, Mt. Selinda, Chivi (Chibi), Masvingo, Gutu, and Chirumhanzu (Chilimanzi). Altogether, there were 448 cases with 67 deaths recorded and 200,000 Africans vaccinated by government officers.[29] Thus attempts to monitor the border contributed to an increase in clandestine crossings which complicated smallpox control efforts.

There were more smallpox outbreaks in Zimbabwe, some of which colonial health officials and Native Commissioners blamed on Africans from Mozambique. However, the most severe outbreaks of smallpox occurred from 1918 to 1922, after which "the mortality rate remained rather insignificant."[30] Yet this declining mortality did little to dampen European settler fears.

Before assessing the African response to smallpox vaccination, it is useful to consider how the colonial officials actually performed vaccinations as this demonstrates the disparity between theory and reality and why there was African opposition to vaccination. The Mozambique Company stated that in order to execute the vaccination, one African auxiliary nurse would accompany an official in charge of the procedure to list the names of individuals vaccinated at each point of visit. This was to be carried out until all the people had been vaccinated or revaccinated.[31]

Authorities in Zimbabwe also provided rules on vaccinations. The Colonial Secretary invoked sections 66 and 81 of the Public Health Act of 1924 to declare a lay vaccinator as any official of the Native (African Affairs) Department, police, or other person whose selection for this service had received approval of the Minister of Health. Every vaccinator

[28] NAZ, A3/12/29: Smallpox, 1910–1922, Letter from the Secretary, Department of Administrator, to the Town Clerk, Salisbury, Rhodesia, 16th January, 1920.

[29] Gelfand, *A Service to the Sick*, 22.

[30] Gelfand, *A Service to the Sick*, 23.

[31] AHM, FCM, Secretaria Geral: Relatórios, Caixa 128, Pasta 2678, Relatório da Direcção dos Serviços de Saúde, 1929: Assistência Sanitaria ao Indígena, 10.

received the following items, which he took with him when proceeding on vaccination duty: a vaccinating needle or lancet, a spirit lamp, and a supply of fresh spirit; and a supply of freshly tested calf lymph in a thermos flask. These articles were supplied as required by the Public Health Department in Harare.

In carrying out vaccination the vaccinator was required to follow the following procedure: to first thoroughly cleanse his hands with warm water, soap and nail brush; thoroughly cleanse the outer side of the upper arm of the person to be vaccinated with soap and water and wipe dry, without using disinfectants; thoroughly sterilize a lancet or vaccinating needle by passing it through the flame of a spirit lamp, or dipping it into boiling water, and then allowing it to cool; and holding the arm of the person to be vaccinated so that the skin of the outer side of the upper arm was kept on the stretch, gently scarify the skin with a number of scratches in three or four separate places. It was important for the vaccinator to warn the person or the parent or guardian, in the case of a child, to avoid washing off the lymph and that the vaccinated area must be kept clean and protected from injury or dirt until the scabs had fallen off. The government ordered the vaccinator to exercise every precaution to ensure scrupulous cleanliness in vaccinating. The vaccinator was also required to sterilize the lancet or needle after vaccinating each person as well as making sure that no lymph was used beyond the date specified on the container.

In addition, the government required every vaccinator to record the names and particulars of every person vaccinated. Also, a record had to be kept of the name and other particulars of every person, and in the case of a child of the parent or guardian declining to be vaccinated and the reason if any, and the same information was to be then transmitted to a magistrate. Moreover, if it came to the knowledge of the vaccinator that any person was suffering from ill effects attributed to vaccination, the vaccinator was required to furnish full particulars including the name and address of the affected person and of his informant, to a magistrate.[32]

By employing laymen as vaccinators, thousands of vaccinations were carried out annually, which would have been impossible if this procedure had been restricted to medical or paramedical personnel only because of their small numbers.[33] The government paid these lay vaccinators for their

[32] NAZ, 1173/357: Public Health Act, 1924–1932, The Government of Southern Rhodesia, Regulations for the performance of vaccination.

[33] Gelfand, *A Service to the Sick*, 21.

services in accordance with guidelines drawn in 1914, which specified three pence per head for the first 100 Africans vaccinated, two pence for up to 200, and one penny for each one above that number.

However, while officials claimed that careful instructions were given to each vaccinator and that "this simple procedure was carried out very successfully,"[34] there is evidence that portrays this procedure as a haphazard one, contributing to African resistance and reluctance to embrace vaccinations. Noel Allison Hunt, who performed vaccinations on Africans in Zimbabwe during the 1920s, explained in 1983, how he performed them,

> Once a year we used to go down and have what we called a vaccination campaign. You *rounded up* all the tribes-people who hadn't been vaccinated. You had a cork with needles in it and one got paid a penny a head (I'd forgotten this, it was a valuable source of income). So[,] one *rounded them up* (with the help of the [African] messengers, of course) and had them in lines of 25 and they all stood there with their left hand on their left hip. First of all[,] a messenger went down with a swab of methylated spirits on cotton wool, cleaned their arms and one then went along and scratched it, [using] the thing with a needle just to get the under skin exposed, the white underskin exposed. Then you went along with the messenger next to you with a handful of these tubes of lymph which you broke and blew on to the sore. *You then told them not to wash it off—which they immediately did, of course.* And off you went. And I can still remember the smell of a Karanga woman's armpit at 2 o'clock on a hot Saturday afternoon, believe me. ... Yeah, well. ... Anyway, for this one got a penny a head.[35]

Phrases, such as "rounded them up," testify to the intrusive nature of such vaccination campaigns on Africans. There exists no data to suggest that the colonial officials requested the consent of Africans or, at least, educated them on why these vaccinations were performed. Neither is there any indication that the vaccination teams singled out the unvaccinated Africans for vaccination in such a military-style vaccination procedure. Many Africans were vaccinated more than once during the colonial period on suspicion of an unsuccessful vaccination whenever there was a smallpox epidemic in their village.

[34] *Ibid.*, 21.

[35] NAZ, ORAL 240: Oral History, Smallpox Vaccination, Interview held with Noel Allison Hunt in England on 27th November, 1983; Interviewer- I. J. Johnstone. Emphasis added.

Also standing out clearly from the aforementioned interview is the fact that African villagers resented such vaccinations as they quickly washed the vaccine from the wounds. This raises questions about the efficacy of these vaccinations. Some Mozambican interviewees said the vaccination exercise was a very unhygienic procedure since the vaccinators used the same cotton swab and needle on everybody without sterilizing the needle. One villager from Muedzwa, Mozambique, Mrs. Chivhovho, recalled that colonial officials forced Africans to submit to vaccination while other Africans fled.[36]

Hunt's account also shows that some members of the vaccination staff regarded the exercise as a money-making venture. As such, compulsory vaccinations served two purposes. One was to conform to the requirements of health officials, and the other one was to earn some money (the more the people vaccinated, the more the money). The tendency to force as many people as possible to be vaccinated to make more money cannot be ruled out completely. This compulsion generated mixed reactions from the African population. Some resisted, others reluctantly submitted.

Also worth noting are some racist connotations in Hunt's story, such as references to a Karanga woman's armpit. Colonial public health officials, too, expressed such racist attitudes, claiming that the "vaccination of natives is a filthy, smelly job which European members of staff object most strongly to performing."[37] High-ranking officials often empathized with European staff involved in vaccinating Africans and suggested that the actual application of vaccines should be done by African clerks.

In Mozambique the vaccination process involved summoning various chiefs to gather people for a vaccination campaign. According to one interviewee, speaking in a group interview,

> The Portuguese would go to the chiefs and summon them to gather their people in one area for the vaccination. They demanded that entire families gather there to be recorded [tying of knots] and vaccinated. The vaccination process could last for a whole week. The Portuguese would go from one headman to another vaccinating people. People had to cook and stay there until the process was completed.[38]

[36] Interview with Mrs. Chivhovho, Muedzwa, Mozambique, December 20, 2006.

[37] Chasokela, "A History of Smallpox in Southern Rhodesia, 1890–1970," 14.

[38] Group interview, Ngaone, Chipinge District, 19 September, 2006. Officials recorded the number of children per household. Tying knots was a way of keeping track of the ages of children, with each knot representing a year. This was done chiefly to determine when a child

Thus, whenever there was a smallpox outbreak, colonial governments took stern public health measures, such as compulsory vaccination as well as surveillance measures to contain the disease. For instance, when an outbreak of smallpox occurred at the end of 1919 in the Mutare District of Zimbabwe, "the vaccination of *all* natives in the district was undertaken and was completed at the end of March [1920]."[39] There were several outbreaks that year, the first at St. Augustine's Mission in February, and the second at Nyamana's "kraal" (village) which culminated in 19 deaths in March 1919. In addition to these two, there were four more outbreaks later that year, one in May at "Park" farm, another one in June at Battery Spruit, and the two more in August at Toronto Mine and on the Mutare Commonage. NC Mutate claimed that in "almost all cases except that of St. Augustine's Mission the sufferers were natives who had recently arrived from Portuguese East Africa."[40]

In Mozambique itself, smallpox continued to be a problem. In its 1929 report on health care for Africans, the Mozambique Company government stated that as far as smallpox prophylaxis was concerned, there was need for compulsory vaccination and the only way to achieve this was to perform a mass vaccination of the whole population using census records.[41]

Twenty-eight years later, in 1948, the NC Mutare repeated his claim that cases of smallpox occurred occasionally, but that these "appeared practically [and] solely amongst alien immigrants from P.E.A. and [had] been reported from the Migrant Labour Depot at Mutasa North Reserve and in Umtali."[42] This reinforced the belief of authorities in colonial Zimbabwe in the diffusion of disease from their Lusophone neighbor and strengthened their resolve to protect Zimbabwe by monitoring the border. However, this also shows how permeable the border was and the

was old enough to be recruited for *zheti* (forced labor). Each adult man had to work for several months on government projects without pay, which was tantamount to slavery. For more on forced labor in central Mozambique, see Eric Allina, *Slavery By Any Other Name: African Life under Company Rule in Colonial Mozambique* (Charlottesville: University of Virginia Press, 2012).

[39] NAZ, S2076: Report of the Native Commissioner, Umtali District for the year ended 31st December 1920. Emphasis added.

[40] *Ibid.*

[41] AHM, FCM, Secretaria Geral: Relatórios, Caixa 128, Pasta 2678, Relatório da Direcção dos Serviços de Saúde, 1929: Assistência Sanitaria ao Indígena, 9–10.

[42] NAZ, S1051: Report of the Native Commissioner, Umtali for the year ended 31st December, 1948.

ineffectiveness of public health policies designed to work along territorial lines in a highly mobile region.

In 1963 after discovering 25 cases of smallpox in the Dora, Zimunya, Chitora, and Penhalonga communal areas, the Mutare City Health Department took some measures to prevent the disease from spreading into the city. These measures consisted of a vaccination campaign from 3 to 5 December, which culminated in the vaccination of 816 Africans. This campaign appeared to bring the disease under control.[43] Two years later another outbreak was recorded in August, which the City of Mutare's Health Department claimed was brought into the city by five Mozambicans from Beira.[44] City officials immediately vaccinated these Mozambicans, but two of them died and a campaign launched during the same month resulted in the vaccination of 4673 Africans. In another smallpox epidemic, a more serious one in September 1971 in Mutare, the city's Health Department launched an extensive house-to-house vaccination campaign in the African townships of Sakubva and Dangamvura from the beginning of November 1971 to the end of January 1972, culminating in the inoculation of over 90 percent of the population.[45] Nevertheless, the question of how African villagers and townsfolk responded to these vaccination campaigns is the subject of the following section.

African Response: Resentment and Resistance

Studies in some parts of colonial Africa have shown that in the early years, when racist stereotypes were stronger, some colonial authorities blamed smallpox outbreaks on African resistance to vaccination, with later references being vague and failure being blamed on low numbers of vaccinations for a given year.[46] These studies have also revealed changes over time in the African reception of vaccinations, from outright refusal to accommodation and demands for public health intervention. The case of colonial Ghana (the Gold Coast) clearly demonstrates this with reports indicating how well and eager Africans were for vaccines, to the extent of

[43] Clever Muyambo, "Medical History of Mutare: A case study of the City's Health Services, 1960–1992," 32.

[44] *Ibid.*

[45] *Ibid.*

[46] Schneider, "The Long History of Smallpox Eradication," 33.

"crying out" for them.[47] Here, the biggest challenge was the ineffectiveness of the vaccines.

While the somewhat similar trends are discernible in the Zimbabwe-Mozambique border region, there is no clear evidence of Africans crying out for vaccinations like in the Gold Coast, except in the case of treatments for sexually transmitted diseases. This shows how this particular community experienced a particularly harsh kind of colonialism and responded in a different way. In the border region of Mozambique and Zimbabwe, therefore, some African villagers and town dwellers reluctantly submitted to vaccination, while others resisted. Resistance to vaccination took many forms, including concealing a smallpox outbreak to avoid vaccination, hiding in the bush to avoid vaccination teams, or even outright refusal to be vaccinated. Commenting on the 1910 smallpox epidemic in Mozambique, the administrator of Macequece expressed disappointment in the way Africans in Manica district responded to smallpox control programs. Although the auxiliary nurse of that district, Joaquim Pedro Fernandes, had inspected the district and recorded morbidity and mortality statistics, this administrator still maintained that the numbers of deaths due to smallpox were more than those obtained by auxiliary Fernandes because the Africans, for fear, hid in the bush and never told the truth.[48]

Interviews carried out in the district of Mossurize confirmed such reactions to smallpox control efforts in Mozambique. In fact, some of the interviewees said that smallpox vaccinations left a permanent scar on the arm. They said that during these years, colonial governments chose different areas of the arm for vaccination. As a result, a person from Mozambique was easily identified by this vaccination mark or scar. Due to the fact that it was the practice of many Africans from Mozambique to go and work in Zimbabwe and particularly in South Africa on the Rand gold mines in Johannesburg, vaccination scars easily exposed them to officials who then deported them if they were illegal immigrants. According to Mr. Muchuchu,

> On smallpox, yes, the Portuguese health officials used to visit villages and vaccinate people against it. The bad thing was that when one went to *Joni*

[47] *Ibid.*

[48] AHM, FCM, Secretaria Geral: Processos, 1892–1942, Epidemias: Varíola e Influenza, Circunscrição de Chimoio. Caixa 131, Pasta 478, Chefe da Circunscrição de Manica-Macequece, para Delegado de Saúde, 17 de Setembro de 1910.

> (Johannesburg, South Africa), South African officials would see the vaccination scar and know that you came from Mozambique. They would then deport you. This vaccination might have been good for disease prevention, but it was bad for work in *Joni*.[49]

Upon their return to their villages in Mozambique, these men often discouraged their children from being vaccinated against smallpox, telling them that vaccination scars would jeopardize their chances of getting relatively better-paying jobs outside Mozambique.

Apart from these marks, Africans also disliked the vaccination process itself. It was often painful and scary because of a prominent wound that sometimes developed on the vaccination spot. According to some interviewees,

> The Portuguese came to perform smallpox vaccinations and after the vaccination a huge wound developed. So, people [Africans] were scared to death that they would die. They could not understand why such a huge wound developed if this was meant to prevent disease. Therefore, as soon as an announcement went out that Portuguese officials were coming to vaccinate, Africans fled, stayed and slept in the bush. Others who did not flee but tried to resist were arrested by the police and forcibly vaccinated.[50]

Some Africans thus could not understand why this process of vaccination resulted in wounds that could endanger their health. Worse still, they sometimes had to go through this process more than once, partly as a result of a failed procedure as the loss of vaccine potency due to heat was an ongoing concern and because of the general rule requiring the vaccination of all people in affected districts.[51]

Similar acts of resistance to vaccination were reported in other parts of Africa—for example, in early colonial Malawi, where "smallpox police" who toured villages and enforced vaccination found it difficult to persuade people that vaccination was beneficial or that it was more effective than their own system of variolation. In the 1919 epidemic, for instance, the smallpox police questioned the system of compulsory vaccination after finding it impossible to prevent widespread evasion because villagers did

[49] Interview with Mr. Muchuchu, Zangiro, Mozambique, 23 September, 2006.
[50] Group Interview, Tanganda Halt, Chipinge District, Zimbabwe, 24 September, 2006.
[51] Schneider, "The Long History of Smallpox Eradication," 28.

not report smallpox cases and women hid their children when smallpox police were in the vicinity.[52]

The implementation of public health policies itself in the villages of Mozambique and Zimbabwe depended on the "cooperation" of African chiefs. Colonial officials punished uncooperative chiefs. In Zimbabwe, for example, all chiefs were required to report smallpox outbreaks. The fate of those who failed to do so was demonstrated by the experience of Chief Nyashanu of Buhera, who failed to report the prevalence of smallpox in his area in 1914 as was required of all chiefs under Section 31, Sub-section 2 of the Southern Rhodesia Native Regulations Proclamation of 1910.[53] Upon being asked why he did not report this epidemic, Chief Nyashanu expressed ignorance of the prevalence of this disease, but public health officials claimed that the disease had been prevalent for six months and among the victims was the chief's own son. To punish the chief for failing to obey smallpox surveillance measures, the government withheld his subsidy for 12 months.

This resistance to vaccination was not confined to the border region. In 1928, for instance, the Native Superintendent who went to supervise smallpox control efforts in Hyde Park encountered acts of resistance. Here, in order to suppress smallpox outbreaks, public health officials resorted to the burning of African villagers' houses, which heightened the sense of grievance inspired by such public health measures. This destruction of houses was in accordance with Part III, Section 41 (m) of the Public Health Act of 1924, which stated that the Minister may make regulations as to,

> the evacuation, closing, alteration or the demolition or destruction of any premises the occupation of which was considered likely to favor the spread or render more difficult the eradication of disease, and the definition of the circumstances under which compensation may be paid in respect of any premises so demolished or destroyed and the manner of fixing such compensation.[54]

While the law made provisions for the payment of compensation by the government, in this Hyde Park case, colonial officials refused to pay for the houses they destroyed in the public health operation. In fact,

[52] Vaughan, *Curing Their Ills*, 43–44. See Feierman, "Struggles for Control," 73–147.
[53] Chasokela, "A History of Smallpox in Southern Rhodesia, 1890–1970," 4.
[54] NAZ, S1173/225-227: Infectious Diseases-Public Health Act, 16.

A. M. Fleming, then the Medical Director said that the government could not compensate for the destruction of property due to smallpox suppression efforts because the infection had occurred due to personal neglect of ordinary precautions and claimed that Africans themselves usually burnt down their houses in three-year intervals for sanitary and other reasons.[55] However, Africans generally destroyed dwellings only when moving considerable distances. No wonder such control measures were unpopular with some Africans.

In addition, during the smallpox outbreak of 1929 in Zimbabwe, which officials claimed had originated in Zambia, Malawi, and Mozambique and spread slowly southward along African routes, reaching the African districts of Mutoko (Mtoko) and Murehwa (Mrewa), these officials said villagers attempted to hide its presence until more than a couple of cases had occurred.[56] After this outbreak was ascertained, public health officials isolated the sick and established cordons of special police. These measures, asserted officials, together with the general vaccination of the African population in the affected areas and in neighboring reserves, "resulted in an early suppression of the epidemic, though some limited outbreaks and sporadic cases continued to occur in other parts of the Colony for some time afterwards."[57]

Furthermore, officials in Zimbabwe monitored the South African border in order to control smallpox. When a smallpox epidemic, thought to have originated from South Africa, occurred in Gwanda, Fort Tuli, and Beitbridge in 1937, public health authorities implemented "exceedingly vigorous measures" after an inspection of the Beitbridge cases revealed that this was an extensive outbreak of virulent smallpox. These measures included the prohibition of the entry of potentially infected persons through Beitbridge until an extensive vaccination barrier had been formed in the area south of a line connecting Bulawayo, Masvingo, and Mutare.[58] However, an inspection of stations along this barrier revealed the existence of some foci of infection in some inaccessible areas at the confluence of the Save and Lundi Rivers. Medical officials noted resistance on the part of Africans in this area, claiming that the Africans' failure to notify authorities

[55] Chasokela, "A History of Smallpox in Southern Rhodesia, 1890–1970," 6.

[56] NAZ, S2419: Reports on Public Health, 1923–1945, Report on the Public Health for the Year 1929, 12.

[57] *Ibid.*, 12–13.

[58] NAZ, S2419: Reports on Public Health, 1923–1945, Report on the Public Health for the Year 1937, 11.

was, in large part, due to the fear that the government would implement repressive measures similar to those which it had enforced during a recent outbreak of foot and mouth disease.[59]

In addition, during the 1948–1952 outbreaks, the vaccination teams encountered enormous difficulties in implementing the vaccination program among the Tonga people of Binga (in Matabeleland, western Zimbabwe) because the Tonga "usually fled at the appearance of vaccination teams."[60] While these cases occurred outside the border region, they help to demonstrate how invasive smallpox control policies were, how widespread the resentment was among Africans, and the "dangers" that the mobility of unvaccinated people supposedly posed to the European settlers.

Within the Zimbabwe-Mozambique border region itself, there were numerous cases of resistance to smallpox control measures. For example, in September 1953, headmen Manjeya, Jairos Mundadi, Sidi, Willie, and Luke of Mutare district, whose duty it was to inform people about vaccination dates and venues, refused, together with their families, to report for vaccination.[61] However, the most prominent cases of resistance came from the African Independent Churches (AICs) during the 1940s and 1950s.

African Independent Churches and Colonial Public Health

As demonstrated in previous chapters, infectious diseases caused much concern among European settlers in both Zimbabwe and Mozambique. This anxiety contributed to intrusive control measures such as compulsory vaccinations, restrictions on African mobility, and an intrusion into African society. Perhaps one of the most disruptive effects of colonial public health was denying some Africans the freedom of assembly and freedom to cross the border for religious purposes from the 1920s onward. This section points to new ways of understanding resistance to colonial rule in Southern Africa by looking at religious opposition to colonial public health initiatives. The result is a broadening the analysis of colonial resistance and oppression beyond the realm of nationalism. Thus while much of the

[59] *Ibid.* Foot and mouth disease control measures included the killing and burning of affected cattle and food stuffs.

[60] Chasokela, "A History of Smallpox in Southern Rhodesia, 1890–1970," 10.

[61] *Ibid.*

recent work on prophetic movements, such as the African Independent Churches (hereafter AICs), rejects the older view that they were essentially anticolonial and proto-nationalist, it remains true that on occasion the prophetic endeavor to cleanse society included attempts to cleanse it of alien and intrusive beliefs and their adherents.[62]

These churches were the Zionist/Apostolic/"VAPOSTORI" or *Mapostori* sects, which resisted medical interventions, including smallpox vaccinations and treatment of diseases on religious grounds. These sects considered vaccination unnatural. In fact, these sects, which had cross-border ties, present a fertile ground for exploring cross-border movements of Africans and disease control. The trans-border nature of these sects is demonstrated by the fact that they commanded a following from both Zimbabwe and Mozambique. There was much cross-border movement to attend church gatherings, heightening colonial officials' fears of smallpox diffusion. These fears led to the implementation of intrusive public health measures.

The Origins and Nature of AICs in Southern Africa

AICs were indigenous in origin and called themselves by words like "Zion," "Apostolic," "Pentecostal," and "Faith."[63] They are also referred to as "Spirit" churches. Historically, they originated from Zion City in Illinois, United States.[64] Ideologically, however, they claim to originate from Mount Zion in Jerusalem, while theologically, scholars consider them to be a syncretic Bantu movement with healing, speaking in tongues, purification rites, and taboos as the main tenets of their faith.[65] It is important to note that whereas the term "Zionist" is commonly used to refer to the advocates of a Jewish homeland, these African "Zionist" churches do not concern themselves with this idea, nor do they have connections with

[62] Terence Ranger, "Plagues of beasts and men," 242.

[63] Bengt Sundkler, *Bantu Prophets in South Africa* (Oxford: Oxford University Press, 1961), 55.

[64] In the early 1900s Zionist missionaries traveled to South Africa and established churches there, with an emphasis on divine healing, abstention from pork, and the wearing of white robes. These were later followed by Pentecostal missionaries who stressed spiritual gifts and baptism in the Holy Spirit, with speaking in tongues being the initial evidence of their teaching.

[65] Sundkler, *Bantu Prophets in South Africa*, 54–55.

Israel.[66] In Southern Africa, these churches sprang out in South Africa and were subsequently spread to Zimbabwe and Mozambique by migrant workers.

These AICs were initially imported to Zimbabwe by migrant workers from Zimbabwe after the First World War when two Ndebele labor migrants, Mabhena and Petrus Ndebele, who had joined the Christian Apostolic Church in South Africa, returned to Matabeleland and began propagating the new faith in the Insiza district.[67] However, their influence beyond Matabeleland was limited. Hence the rise of the Zionist movement among the Shona of the Mozambique-Zimbabwe border region can be traced to the 1920s when Mtisi, a Ndau migrant worker from Chipinge introduced the Zionist church from South Africa. Mtisi was among the first of the Shona leaders to join the South African Zionists in 1921.[68] He was also the first of the Shona Zionist evangelists to return to Zimbabwe, and upon his return, he started preaching in the Chipinge district from his homestead called "Zion City."

In terms of their beliefs and practices, these churches were sometimes referred to as churches of prophecy, healing, and the Holy Spirit.[69] It is precisely due to their belief in faith healing that these churches were opposed to any kind of medical intervention. For this reason, they should not be confused with some Pentecostal churches in Zimbabwe and Mozambique which encourage the use of Western biomedicine.

The importance of healing in Zionist churches helps to explain why they were against medical intervention. The Tshidi of South Africa, for example, offer invaluable insights on this subject. The mushrooming of distinct movements, collectively known as "Zionist" or "Spirit" churches, among them was based on a range of inspired leaders who were conceived of as healers rather than ministers as is the case in the Protestant mold.[70] The centrality of faith healing contributed to the resistance to colonial public health initiatives such as smallpox vaccination. This healing was not

[66] Terence Ranger, "African Initiated Churches," *Transformation* 24, 2 (2007): 65.

[67] M. L. Daneel, *Old and New in the Southern Shona Independent Churches, Volume I: Background and Rise of the Major Movements* (The Hague: Mouton and Co., 1971), 286.

[68] *Ibid.*, 288.

[69] *Ibid.*, 66.

[70] Jean Comaroff, *Body of Power, Spirit of Resistance: The Culture and History of a South African People* (Chicago: University of Chicago Press, 1985), 166.

only for physical ailments. It was holistic.[71] Thus while these churches varied in socio-cultural form, the majority of them were multipurpose associations, organized around a focal ritual place and a holistic ideological scheme. They were full of energy and creativity and emphasized the ritual reconstruction of the body through rites of healing, dietary taboos, and carefully prescribed uniforms.[72] Healing was so central to these churches to the extent that they have been referred to as "medico-religious social movements."[73]

As a result of their grounding in faith healing, any attempt by colonial health officials to enforce public health measures threatened the very basis of the existence of such churches and also threatened to usurp the position of the church leader as the chief healer. One interviewee recalled that colonial officials prohibited Apostolic gatherings "because they thought these gatherings would spread smallpox, but the Apostolic leaders argued that nothing could happen at these gatherings because they had prophesied about them."[74] Church members refused medicine saying Jesus Christ did not move around with medicines.[75] Another interviewee said that the *Mapostori* even refused purified or treated water because they believed that there were chemicals in that water, which they took to be medicine.[76] Instead, the *Mapostori* blessed and drank their own water (holy water), which they believed could heal the sick. This demonstrates that the *Mapostori* placed more faith in their prophecies than in public health measures. Accepting medical interventions such as smallpox vaccinations was thus tantamount to doubting the validity of their prophecies and their faith.

In addition, Apostolic beliefs accorded better with older ideas about the causation of disease than did European vaccination campaigns. These older ideas attributed some diseases to evil spirits and misfortune, which to the *Mapostori*, needed divine intervention. The *Mapostori* believed that witchcraft was real and "treated" patients who they thought had been

[71] Ezra Chitando, "Spirit-Type Churches as Holistic Healing Movements: A Study of the Johane Masowe WeChishanu Church," B.A. Honors Dissertation, Department of Religious Studies, Classics and Philosophy, University of Zimbabwe, 1991, 6.

[72] Comaroff, *Body of Power, Spirit of Resistance, 167.*

[73] Harold W. Turner, *African Independent Church, Volume II: The life and faith of the Church of the Lord (Aladura)* (Oxford: Clarendon Press, 1967), 108.

[74] Interview, Nyamakamba Village, Zimunya District, Mutare South, Zimbabwe, 31 July, 2006.

[75] Interview, Mvududu Village, Mutare South, Zimbabwe, 1 August, 2006.

[76] Interview, Chitakatira Village, Mutare South, Zimbabwe, 31 July, 2006.

bewitched while encouraging Shona beliefs in ancestral spirits and practices such as polygamy. Consulting Western medical practitioners was a breach of fundamental church doctrine and resulted in excommunication from the church. Hence, the punishment for visiting clinics and hospitals often involved the church's refusal to bury church members who died at clinics or hospitals. However, those who used Western medicine could be forgiven if they confessed their sins. The church could welcome them back to the fellowship.[77]

Some scholars have theorized that the publication of Christian scriptures in indigenous languages contributed to the rise of AICs.[78] As Africans began to discern the scriptures, they noted discrepancies between missionary teaching and biblical teaching in areas such as family, land, fertility, and the significance of women, and thought the Bible endorsed polygamy and respect for ancestors.[79] Thus, the dearth of understanding and sometimes austere rules of the missionaries with regard to polygamy, the use of beer, and ancestor worship were responsible for the way that the African members of the mission churches broke away and joined up with the AICs.[80] Early AICs therefore adopted and intensified missionary evangelicalism with a quest to Christianize African tradition far more profoundly than the missionaries and their catechists had been able to do.[81]

AICs and Colonial Public Health

AICs presented the most coordinated and formidable resistance to colonial public health initiatives. For some of these AICs, opposition to the border public health became the main method of resisting colonial rule. While these sects emerged out of African interactions with the Western church, the apparent ease with which Africans internalized the principles of the Western church camouflaged an often vigorous resistance to the

[77] Interview, Zangiro, Mozambique, 23 September, 2006.

[78] David B. Barrett, *Schism and Renewal in Africa: An Analysis of Six Thousand Contemporary Religious Movements* (Nairobi: Oxford University Press, 1968), 268.

[79] *Ibid.*

[80] M. L. Daneel, *Zionism and Faith-Healing in Rhodesia: Aspects of African Independent Churches* (The Hague: Mouton and Co, 1970), 11.

[81] Terence O. Ranger, "Introduction," in *Evangelical Christianity and Democracy in Africa*, ed. Terence O. Ranger (Oxford: Oxford University Press, 2006), 6. See also Terence Ranger, "Taking on the Missionary's Task: African Spirituality and the Mission Churches of Manicaland in the 1930s," *Journal of Religion in Africa* 29, 2 (1999): 175–205.

culture of colonial domination.[82] In Zimbabwe, the comparatively late emergence of AICs among the Shona was a result of many factors, such as the strict control on movements of sectarian preachers by the government.[83]

Although these AICs have featured prominently in the narrative of anti-colonial "resistance history," it has been argued that they played an ambiguous part because they "were usually aloof from and sometimes actively at odds with the secular nationalist movements."[84] This ambiguity, however, should be examined within the scope of their most heartfelt concerns. For these movements, the intrusion of health and healing space was the most important grievance against colonial rule.

In Mozambique, as in other parts of Southern and Central Africa, AICs offered an opportunity for laborers and peasants to vent their hostility against the new social order and what they considered to be the hypocrisy of the established Christian churches. As indicated in a report prepared by the Portuguese secret police, the popularity of the separatist churches was due to both the racial discrimination within the colonies and the lack of sensitivity on the part of the European missionaries with regard to Africans.[85] Thus colonial officials considered the activities of these sects to be acts of insubordination to colonial authority.

From their very inception in Zimbabwe, the Zionist/Apostolic sects attracted the attention of colonial authorities, particularly Native Commissioners. In 1932, for instance, the NC Chipinge wrote in his annual report under the section "Political Situation" that,

> Of political activity in the customary sense of that word there has been little or nothing, nothing at least that has been sufficiently public to reach my ears. … Nevertheless, there has of late been a feeling in the air, so to speak, of what one might, perhaps, best call insubordination, emanating undoubtedly from scattered numbers of local Natives who had some schooling here before they made their traditional journeys to the Johannesburg mines. It is a feeling never openly expressed but often obliquely voiced in the course of

[82] *Ibid.*, 19.

[83] T. O. Ranger, "The Early history of Independency in Rhodesia," in *Religion in Africa: proceedings of a seminar held in the Centre of African Studies*, University of Edinburgh, 10th–12th April, 1964.

[84] Ranger, "Introduction," 9. See also Terence Ranger, "Religious Movements and Politics in sub-Saharan Africa," *African Studies Review* 29, 2 (1986): 1–69.

[85] Isaacman and Isaacman, *Mozambique*, 72.

> prayers and local preachings by way of metaphor and parable. ... The discontented Natives tend to look heavenwards for the change they desire from their earthly condition which they have come to believe has been unjustly imposed upon them by the whites. At first, therefore, we hear only whisperings and prayers, later we may see open defiance and attempts at direct hostility.[86]

The NC clearly expressed his discomfort in the activities of church members coming from work in Johannesburg, South Africa. Also glaring was the AICs' preoccupation with religion as a way of expressing their dislike of colonial rule.

On the Mozambican side of the border, almost all independent churches traced their origins to separatist church movements (Zionist and Ethiopian) in neighboring South Africa and Zimbabwe.[87] Mozambican migrant laborers had found refuge in these churches while in South Africa and Zimbabwe, and when they returned home, they either formed branches or founded autonomous sects fashioned after their South African and Zimbabwean counterparts.[88] This in itself is evidence of the transnational nature of these churches, drawing a following from various colonies and posing what, in the eyes of colonial officials, were "threats" to public health as these churches resisted vaccination or any medical intervention, whether Western or "traditional."

In Zimbabwe in 1932, the NC Chipinge wrote that toward the end of that year, reports reached him "of certain ebulliences in the form of continuous night-dancing of both sexes conducted by the local leader [of an Apostolic sect], one Jeremiah."[89] The NC thus called for a meeting in the Mutema Reserve at which he "enjoined the reputed members of this sect to discontinue entirely those objectionable practices." In fact, this NC had spoken with a prophetic voice when he hinted that "later we may see open defiance and attempts at direct hostility" because the 1940s and 1950s witnessed such open defiance against smallpox vaccinations. In 1948, for instance, nurses at Nyanyadzi clinic treated a young smallpox patient,

[86] NAZ, S235/510 Native Commissioners Reports: Report of the Native Commissioner for the Melsetter District, for the Year ended 31st December, 1932.

[87] Isaacman and Isaacman, *Mozambique*, 72.

[88] *Ibid.*

[89] NAZ, S235/510 Native Commissioners Reports: Report of the Native Commissioner for the Melsetter District, for the Year ended 31st December, 1932. Mutema, Nyanyadzi, and, in fact, the entire area under the Melsetter District were inside the border region.

whose parents, being members of the Apostolic Church in Marange (Maranke) Communal Land, refused to have their children vaccinated. This Apostolic sect was the most prominent in the Zimbabwe-Mozambique border region, led by Johane Marange from the Marange Communal Land in the Mutare district.

Despite the resistance to vaccination among sect members in Zimbabwe, there was, according to colonial officials in Zimbabwe, an added danger in that these churches drew congregants from the supposedly diseased and poorly governed Mozambique Company territory. A report by the Rhodesian Criminal Investigation, for instance, indicated that one of the *Mapostori* church preachers, Takawira, had gone to Johannesburg to preach "accompanied by an unknown native stated to be the representative of the sect in Portuguese East Africa."[90] The NC Mutare had also reported in 1946 that an Apostolic meeting that took place in his district inside the border region was attended by approximately 1000 men, women, and children, "drawn from the Salisbury, Darwin, Hartley, Gwanda, Mazoe [Mazowe], Buhera, Chipinge, Makoni, Marandellas [Marondera] and Umtali districts plus a few from Portuguese Territory and a few other aliens."[91] One elder indicated that members of this religious sect often crossed the border into Mozambique, traveling over 60 miles to as far as Machaze in the border region for their gatherings.[92]

These religious gatherings continued to command a following from across the southern and eastern borders of Zimbabwe. For instance, in 1952, while proceeding to the southern section of the Marange Reserve for a vaccination campaign which had been arranged in conjunction with the Native Department, the Health Inspector was informed by one of the lay vaccinators of a gathering of members of the Apostolic church in the Reserve. The lay vaccinator indicated that the *Mapostori* had gathered there for two weeks and that "representatives from as far afield as Salisbury, Gwelo, Bulawayo, and Johannesburg were attending and were 'too many' in number."[93]

[90] NAZ, S2810/2337; Criminal Investigation Department, Rhodesia—Mapostles, and Apostoles "Johanne," 24th July 1946.

[91] NAZ, S2810/2337: Mapostles, and Apostoles "Johanne," Letter from the Provincial Native Commissioner, Umtali, to the Chief Native Commissioner, Salisbury, 14th August, 1946.

[92] Interview, Harare, Zimbabwe, 24 July, 2006.

[93] NAZ, S2810/2337: Vaccination Campaign—Maranke Reserve, Letter from the Regional Health Inspector, Eastern, Umtali, to the Native Commissioner, Umtali and the Director of Preventative Services, 23rd July, 1952.

However, by the time the Health Inspector arrived at the camping site, the meeting had ended and vehicles were already transporting the attendees from the site. The Inspector estimated that only about 750 people were still at the site. He then asked the chief of the area for permission to vaccinate the people and the chief agreed because it was a government order. While the chief appeared to be understanding, the Inspector claimed that the same could not be said of the other adherents because as the reason for his visit became known, "people started running to the four corners of the compass" in an act of resistance to vaccination.

As the Inspector recalled, when "an attempt was made to form the usual vaccination lines other people in apparent paroxysms of grief jostled the line and continually broke it up." He added, "[w]ithin about 15 minutes, some 400–500 crazy, head wagging, half-demented, singing and screaming lunatics were raging up and down, surrounding the lorry [truck] and generally impeding the course of an efficient vaccination campaign."[94] It was at this point that the Inspector felt it "politic to retire, if not in confusion with dishonour." His African lay vaccinators informed him that if he had not been present, these *Mapostori* would have harmed them. As shown above, Africans who worked with colonial health officials as lay vaccinators were particularly in danger of retaliatory attacks. They were on the frontlines, working as cultural brokers and mediators.[95]

During the same year, in an attempt to stop cross-border attendance at such religious gatherings in African reserves, colonial officials in Zimbabwe invoked Sub-section 1 of Section 42 of the Rhodesian constitution, which stated that the Native Reserves were set apart for the sole and exclusive use by and occupation of the indigenous (African) inhabitants of the colony. Colonial officials also relied on the Settlement of Colonial Natives in Native Kraals Prohibition Act, which prohibited the settlement of "colonial natives" in "native kraals" in Zimbabwe.[96] In addition, Section 3 of the Prevention of Trespass (Native Reserves) Act prohibited the entry of non-indigenous Africans into African reserves. Hence, colonial officials

[94] *Ibid.*

[95] For a detailed discussion of the role of intermediaries and subordinates, see Ryan Johnson and Amna Khalid, ed., *Public Health in the British Empire: Intermediaries, Subordinates, and the Practice of Public Health, 1850–1960* (Routledge: New York, 2012).

[96] NAZ, S2810/2337: "Native Affairs Act (Chapter 72): Section 51" "Lawful of Reasonable Order," 1952. "Colonial natives" were Africans from other British colonies, such as Nyasaland and Northern Rhodesia.

declared, "*Alien natives will not be invited to enter the Reserves for the purpose of attending these [Mapostori] meetings.*"[97] Colonial officials claimed that the presence of large numbers of Africans from other colonies in the reserves spread infection and were concerned as they believed that infectious diseases spread from the African reserves to European areas. They also believed that the presence of huge numbers of "alien natives" increased acts of insubordination as these foreigners were not bound by Zimbabwean laws. There were several African reserves in the border region, set aside for the sole occupation by indigenous Africans. These included the Musikavanhu, Mutema, Ngorima, Muusha, Ndowoyo, Zimunya, Marange, Mutasa, and Jenya. The colonial government later renamed them Tribal Trust Lands in the 1960s.

While efforts were underway to prohibit the cross-border movements of AIC members, resistance from within Zimbabwe continued. The NC Mutare reported in 1952 that vaccination in Jenya, Marange, Zimunya, and Mutasa reserves had continued throughout the year despite some opposition from "VAPOSTORI."[98] The NC added that some of the "VAPOSTORI" were prosecuted and eventually the others fell in line. In 1956 the NC Chipinge, south of Mutare, reported that due to continuous routine vaccination, with 9843 people having been vaccinated that year, there were no cases of smallpox, but three villagers "were prosecuted for refusing, because of alleged religious scruples, to submit to vaccination."[99]

Due to such acts of resistance emanating from Zionist/Apostolic churches, medical officials came to regard the members of these sects as reservoirs of smallpox. Officials also began mulling over some legislation to prohibit church meetings if the members did not submit to vaccination. In fact, this thinking reflected the tendency within colonial circles to blame Africans for the introduction of epidemics into European enclaves. In Zimbabwe, for instance, the Minister of Internal Affairs had claimed that, almost every year, there came from the reserves "epidemics of small-pox, chicken-pox, whooping cough and mumps, some of which affect the

[97] *Ibid.* Emphasis added.

[98] NAZ S2403/268: Annual Report of the Native Commissioner, Umtali for the year ended 31st December, 1952.

[99] NAZ, S2827/2/2/4: Report of the Native Commissioner, Chipinga, for the year ending 31st December, 1956.

children of Europeans, interfere with their educational progress, and tax the capacity of the Health Department of the country to suppress."[100]

Colonial officials therefore started to draft some laws regarding vaccination of members of the AICs at their annual gatherings because of the outbreaks of smallpox they argued were linked to these sects. The NC Mutare, for instance, recorded an extensive outbreak of smallpox in August and September of 1958, which he claimed, was traced back to a large meeting of the Apostolic Sect in the Marange Reserve.[101] The nature of this outbreak was "fortunately mild," but the disease was carried to several districts before the Department of Health contained it. As a result of a meeting between health authorities and leading members of the Apostolic and Zionist sects in the border region, "it was agreed that while the latter would not positively commit their members to vaccination, any proposal to hold meetings of any size would be notified in advance so that protective measures could be undertaken where considered necessary."[102]

Thus on October 31, 1958, D. A. W. Rittey, Director of Medical Services, wrote to the Secretary for Health, "as you are aware, we have had considerable difficulty all over the territory in vaccinating the religious sects Apostolic/Zionist owing to their religious objections," and that as a result, there were outbreaks of smallpox directly traceable to gatherings of this sect, particularly in the Marange Reserve.[103] Rittey suggested that Section 41 of the Public Health Act of 1924 should be invoked to prohibit Zionist/Apostolic church meetings on grounds of public health.[104]

In order to solve this Zionist/Apostolic sect problem, Rittey presented suggestions from various officials. These included vaccinating all people attending Apostolic rallies, which Rittey himself did not favor. Such methods, he believed, would lead to "forcible vaccination, and since these gatherings often number several thousands" there was a serious risk of provoking public disturbance, resulting in the failure to vaccinate. The other suggestion was to ensure that all persons attending these rallies were

[100] NAZ, S2419: Report on the Public Health for the Year 1938, 8.

[101] NAZ, S2827/2/2/6: Annual Report of the Native Commissioner, Umtali, for the Year ended 31st December, 1958.

[102] *Ibid.*

[103] NAZ, F122/400/7/31: Smallpox, 1955–1961, D. A. W. Rittey, The Director of Medical Services (Southern Rhodesia), to D. M. Blair, Secretary for Health, 31st October, 1958.

[104] NAZ, F122/FH/30/15: Smallpox, 1955–1959, D. A. W. Rittey, Director of Medical Services, to the Secretary for Health, 19th November, 1958.

vaccinated before the gathering took place. This meant that colonial officials would deny permission for religious gatherings unless all the attendees were vaccinated.[105] Rittey indicated that there was the possibility that the organizers of the rallies might refuse to accept these conditions and therefore suggested that these measures could be enforced by the Public Health Act under Section 41 (a), (c), and (d). This section of the Public Health Act gave the Minister of Health powers to make regulations, in the case of the occurrence or threatened outbreak of any formidable epidemic disease, to restrict activities, such as gatherings or meetings for the purpose of public worship.[106] This meant that the Minister of Health had extraordinary powers under the Public Health Act to interfere with religious observance.

Furthermore, on November 6, 1958, D. M. Blair, then Secretary for Health, in support of Rittey, claimed that any large meetings of persons who were not vaccinated against smallpox constituted a danger to public health.[107] He asserted that there was "ample evidence in Southern Rhodesia that religious rallies of such nature have often been followed by widespread outbreaks of smallpox by unvaccinated incubating cases of the disease *travelling far and wide*."[108] It was true that these gatherings drew followers from many parts of the border region, including from Mozambique. One interviewee said that the *Mapostori* refused to cancel their gatherings because they "had invited people from distant places."[109] The *Mapostori* therefore could not just tell their followers to go back. They continued with their plans and the police would come to watch over.

However, this practice of police just coming to "watch over" ended when colonial officials devised ways of forcing the *Mapostori* to undergo smallpox vaccinations. Blair favored the proposition of the Secretary for Native Affairs, that is, enforcing vaccination or canceling the gathering in case of noncompliance, and did not see any reason why action could not be taken as an emergency measure in terms of Section 76 of the Public Health Act (Chapter 140) if the organizers of the meeting did not cooperate. Blair added that under the Public Health Act, the Provincial Medical

[105] *Ibid.*

[106] *Ibid.*

[107] NAZ, F122/400/7/31: Smallpox, 1955–1961, D. M. Blair, Secretary for Health, to The Director of Medical Services (Southern Rhodesia), 6th November, 1958.

[108] *Ibid.* Emphasis added.

[109] Interview, Nyamakamba Village, Zimunya, Mutare South, Zimbabwe, 31 July, 2006.

Officer of Health could seek a Ministerial instruction to enforce disease control measures.[110]

All these suggestions demonstrate that there was much debate among government officials about Zionist/Apostolic sects. Responding to the aforementioned suggestions, T. G. Osler, Provincial Medical Officer of Health for the eastern districts of Zimbabwe, said that he did not wish to vaccinate *all* people attending these apostolic rallies "*as the Apostolics have in the past caused disturbances and threatened assaults to the Vaccinators, who would then have to run away, leaving the Apostolics masters of the situation.*"[111] Rittey ended the debate by ordering "no vaccination/no meetings and this continues until you [Zionists/Mapostori] come to your senses."[112]

Yet even these laws and prosecutions did not deter these sects. In what appeared to be a classic case of concealing smallpox cases, in February 1959, soon after the notification of a smallpox case at the Birchenough

[110] NAZ, F122/400/7/31: Smallpox, 1955–1961, D. M. Blair, Secretary for Health, to The Director of Medical Services (Southern Rhodesia), 6th November, 1958. Section 76 of the Public Health Act, 1924 (emergency vaccination of population in areas threatened with smallpox) stated that in the event of the occurrence or threatened occurrence outbreak of smallpox in any area (1) the local authority or its medical officer of health or the government medical officer may require any person to be forthwith vaccinated or revaccinated who has or is suspected to have been in any way recently exposed to smallpox infection or may require the parent or guardian of any child who has or is suspected to have been so exposed to have such child vaccinated or revaccinated forthwith. Any person failing to comply with such requirement shall be guilty of an offence; (2) the local authority may, or when instructed by the Minister so to do shall, require all persons or specified classes of persons within an area defined to attend at centers according to instructions issued and to undergo inspection, vaccination or revaccination as circumstances may require. Such instructions may be issued by notice in the Press or by notices posted in public places or otherwise as may be deemed sufficient by the local authority. Non-attendance shall be deemed to be an offence; (3) any government medical officer, public vaccinator, or medical practitioner duly authorized by the Minister or the local authority may require any person in such area to furnish satisfactory proof (including the exhibition of vaccination scars) that he has been successfully vaccinated within five years immediately preceding the date of such requirement. Any person who fails to furnish such proof as regards himself or as regards any child of which he is the parent or guardian, and refuses to allow himself or such child to be vaccinated, shall be guilty of an offence.

[111] NAZ, F122/400/7/31: Smallpox, 1955–1961, T. G. Osler, Provincial Medical Officer of Health, Eastern, to D. A. W. Rittey, Director of Medical Services, 14th November, 1958. Emphasis added.

[112] NAZ, F122/400/7/31: Smallpox, 1955–1961, D. A. W. Rittey, Director of Medical Services, to the Secretary for Health, 19th November, 1958.

Bridge clinic, the Government Health Inspector (GHI) for Chipinge District proceeded to Headman Zvenyika's area, with three Native (African) Lay Vaccinators (NLVs), ready to vaccinate villagers in the Magetsi area where they thought the outbreak had originated. However, right from the beginning they encountered strong opposition, mostly in the form of passive resistance, as "No one, including the Headman, knew where Magetsi kraal [village] was. No one ever heard of the patient's father, Nyamasana."[113] The villagers claimed they had never heard of any smallpox or any disease remotely resembling smallpox and claimed that there had been no deaths for several months. Yet the GHI heard the direct opposite of the above from storekeepers and teachers, who told him that there were several deaths, but could not give definite information. In fact, there were several smallpox cases in the villages of at least four headmen, Makumbo, Zvenyika, Matudzi, and Muzirikayi. In order to get to these cases, the GHI reported,

> We then got hold (literally) of the Headman Matudsi [Matudzi] and gently persuaded him to show us some smallpox cases. He took us for a distance of about seven miles over the worst possible terrain to three chicken pox cases, laughing up his sleeve as he very well knew that they were not smallpox. By this time the sun had set and it was late when we returned to Matudsi's kraal. The following morning we accidentally discovered that the N. C. Buhera, was nearby at a place called Msasa. … I explained our difficulty to him, [the N. C., Mr Reed] that I get no co-operation from the people, presumably because they are almost a 100 [percent] Zionists and Apostoles, including the Chief, Ny[a]shanu and his Headmen, also that I noted very few vaccination marks on the arms of children that should have been vaccinated.[114]

This was another clear case of resistance from Zionist/Apostolic sects. However, the GHI and his team eventually managed to examine 295 children who should have been vaccinated, only to find that 203 (that is, 68.8

[113] NAZ, F122/400/7/31: Smallpox, 1955–1961, The Government Health Inspector, Chipinga, to The Provincial Medical Officer of Health (Eastern), Umtali, 23rd February, 1959. The Birchenough Bridge area covers both the eastern (in Chipinge District) and western banks of the Save River. The eastern bank falls into the border region, but the Birchenough Bridge clinic (now hospital) was located on the western bank of the Save. This clinic served Africans from both banks of the Save.

[114] *Ibid.*

percent!) had no vaccination marks. Two NLVs then remained in the area to vaccinate these children as the GHI left for Chipinge.

However, the period from May 1959 onward witnessed the application of Rittey's order. The organizers of Apostolic church gatherings had to first apply for permission, indicating the number of people expected, where these people would come from, and the duration of the gatherings. They were also required by law to agree to have their church members inspected by public health officials as well as agreeing to the vaccination of the unvaccinated. Public health officials turned down some of these applications on grounds of public health. In May 1959, for instance, T. G. Osler informed Rittey regarding a proposed African Apostolic gathering scheduled for July 8–18, 1959, in Marange, to which persons were expected from all parts of Zimbabwe. The organizer of this gathering, Johane, expected approximately 800–1000 attendees. Osler prohibited the proposed meeting saying that "there was [the] threat of spread of smallpox from [the neighboring districts of] Buhera, Bikita, Zaka."[115] He added that with such a large number of persons spread about the area for ten days, public health officials were not sure if they could inspect all attendees and vaccinate those requiring a vaccination and that public health officials could not visit all cases of illness suspected to be smallpox.

Johane then asked for a local gathering in Marange in July, with fewer people attending, but Osler reiterated that the case would be considered on its merits, only to be allowed if public health officials could carry out the necessary inspections and vaccinations. Osler said that public health officials would require the meeting not to last longer than two to three days, that the people to attend the gathering should be local to Marange, that the number of persons attending "should not be excessive" from his point of view, and that the organizer would have to require all attendees to comply with public health precautions.[116] Clearly, smallpox control efforts interfered with the regular church activities of the Zionist sects. Implicit in Osler's aforementioned statements was also the cross-border appeal of AIC gatherings because colonial officials were concerned that these religious gatherings generally drew people and allegiance from the supposedly diseased and poorly governed Mozambique.

[115] NAZ, F122/400/7/31: Smallpox, 1955–1961, T. G. Osler, Provincial Medical Officer of Health, Eastern, to D. A. W. Rittey, Director of Medical Services, 6th May, 1959.

[116] *Ibid.*

Another method employed by colonial public health officials to prevent spread of smallpox involved the setting up of road blocks or check points on major routes leading to AIC gathering places. Here officials ordered all pedestrians to disembark and submit to inspection and smallpox vaccination for those not vaccinated. One interviewee who used to be a bus driver remembered,

> At one time, there was a Mapostori gathering in Buhera [on the west bank of the Save, outside the border region]. The police established road block on all roads leading to this gathering, including on the road crossing the Save River. I was transporting Mapostori to the Buhera, across the Save [from the east]. When we reached the roadblock, the police forced the Mapostori to be vaccinated. Women and children bowed to the pressure, but the men refused and fled. They later used bush paths in order to get to the meeting place in Buhera.[117]

Colonial officials had many reasons to monitor or even prohibit such meetings. The members of these religious groups often gathered for weeks, reported officials, without any suitable sanitary provisions, no proper toilets or safe drinking water, and they often resorted to cutting down trees for firewood and to construct temporary shelters. Colonial officials felt the need to intervene and interfere with the activities of these religious groups.

Eventually, however, some bowed to colonial pressures. For example, the Provincial Health Inspector in charge of a "kraal to kraal" vaccination of the whole of Marange Reserve in 1959 claimed that he had received "a great deal of co-operation" from all villagers, including members of the African Apostolic Faith.[118] The NC Mutare then noted, "it would seem that even the most unenlightened Africans now appreciate the benefit of protection against smallpox."[119]

However, others refused to surrender. For them, the intrusion of health and healing space became the most important grievance against colonial rule. This attitude has even survived the dismantling of colonialism. In Zimbabwe, for instance, these AICs have been considered to be "schools of democracy," that is, avenues for the education of otherwise voiceless

[117] Interview, Chitakatira Village, Mutare South, Zimbabwe, July 31, 2006.

[118] NAZ, S2827/2/2/7: Annual Report of the Native Commissioner, Umtali, for the Year ended 31st December, 1959.

[119] *Ibid.*

Zimbabweans in the norms and practices of participatory politics because they promote democracy through the Christian ideals of love, peace, and harmony as they seek to oppose political injustice.[120]

Conclusion

Due to their intrusive nature, public health policies implemented against smallpox triggered mixed reactions from Africans, including accommodation but most importantly resistance, which manifested itself in many forms. For some Africans, such as those belonging to AICs, opposition to vaccination became one of the ways of confronting colonialism. This represents a departure from the traditional historiography of the anticolonial struggle, which emphasizes nationalism.

In addition, as the other chapters have shown, the fear of contagion among European settlers contributed to the implementation of intrusive public health policies. That smallpox was a highly contagious disease amplified these fears, leading to prohibition of worship and restrictions on African mobility. Colonial public health campaigns therefore threatened the basis of some African beliefs and it was not surprising that there was so much resistance to them. This African resistance to colonial public health was also a way of questioning the legitimacy of the colonial state.

Smallpox was therefore one of the world's most feared diseases until a collaborative global vaccination program led by the World Health Organization (hereafter WHO) eradicated the disease in 1980. According to the WHO, the last recorded natural case of smallpox occurred in Somalia in 1977.[121] After this outbreak, the only known cases resulted from a laboratory accident in 1978 in Birmingham, England, which killed one person and caused a limited epidemic.[122] In general, however, the eradication of smallpox was never an easy endeavor. Even the WHO's concerted efforts encountered resistance, prompting the WHO to resort to coercion in other parts of the world such as South Asia.[123]

[120] Isabel Mukonyora, "Foundations for Democracy in Zimbabwe's Evangelical Christianity," in Terence O. Ranger (ed.) *Evangelical Christianity and Democracy in Africa* (Oxford: Oxford University Press, 2008), 136.

[121] World Health Organization, "Health Topics: Smallpox," https://www.who.int/csr/disease/smallpox/en/, accessed on October 13, 2019.

[122] *Ibid.*

[123] See Paul Greenough, "Intimidation, coercion and resistance in the final stages of the South Asian Smallpox Eradication Campaign, 1973–1975," *Social Science and Medicine* 41,

While smallpox has now been eradicated worldwide, it is important to note that this took a concerted effort from the WHO and international cooperation, which was difficult to achieve between Zimbabwe and Mozambique. Smallpox outbreaks in the Zimbabwe-Mozambique border region continued well into the 1970s.[124] It was not until 1977 that the WHO's International Commission for Smallpox Eradication certified smallpox eradication in Mozambique, together with Tanzania, Zambia, and Malawi.[125]

By focusing on smallpox epidemics in the Zimbabwe-Mozambique border region, this chapter has demonstrated that cross-border movements, whether transnational or internal, affected the epidemiology of diseases. Colonial officials in Zimbabwe often claimed that these movements contributed greatly to the difficulties in eradicating smallpox in the region and monitored the border in order to safeguard their health. While the border itself became an obstacle to the control and eradication of smallpox, diffusion of disease from other colonies was not the only reason for smallpox outbreaks. The British in colonial Zimbabwe exaggerated rates of diffusion from Mozambique due to their prejudice against the Portuguese and sometimes to mask the futility of their own interventions.

It is by no coincidence, however, that in both Mozambique and Zimbabwe, the last recorded cases of smallpox occurred in the late 1970s.[126] Arbitrary colonial boundaries which divided people of common origins and culture meant that control and eradication of smallpox was a difficult exercise partly due to occasional diffusion of this disease through cross-border movements as infectious diseases respect no boundaries. Thus, while colonial authorities dealt with outbreaks they believed were brought in by immigrants, they often failed to acknowledge outbreaks

5 (1995): 633–45. In other parts of Asia, such as Cambodia, it was the use of lower caste people in producing the vaccine through the arm to arm technique which caused problems among the upper castes. See Sokhieng Au, *Mixed Medicines: Health and Culture in French Colonial Cambodia* (Chicago: University of Chicago Press, 2011).

[124] Chasokela, "A History of Smallpox in Southern Rhodesia, 1890–1970," 17, O. Ransford, *Bid the Sickness Cease: Disease in the History of Black Africa* (London: John Murray Publishers, 1983), 211. See also Muyambo, "Medical History of Mutare," 32.

[125] AHM, Saúde, Boletim a Saúde em Moçambique, Caixa no. 22, 1978, Pasta no.12.

[126] NAZ, RG-P/FOR 35 Health Services and Mortality Statistics in Rhodesia and other African Countries, Fact Paper 4/77 and AHM, Saúde, Boletim a Saúde em Moçambique, Caixa no. 104, Pasta no. 36, 1979, 10. See also Muyambo, "Medical History of Mutare," 32.

from local foci of infections among those who refused to be vaccinated. Either way, the border was still central in the conception and implementation of public health policy.

References

Au, Sokhieng. *Mixed Medicines: Health and Culture in French Colonial Cambodia*. Chicago: University of Chicago Press, 2011.

Barrett, David B. *Schism and Renewal in Africa: An Analysis of Six Thousand Contemporary Religious Movements*. Nairobi: Oxford University Press, 1968.

Chasokela, F. "A History of Smallpox in Southern Rhodesia, 1890–1970." B. A. Honors Dissertation, Department of History, University of Zimbabwe, 1985.

Chitando, Ezra. "Spirit-Type Churches as Holistic Healing Movements: A Study of the Johane Masowe WeChishanu Church." B.A. Honors Dissertation, Department of Religious Studies, Classics and Philosophy, University of Zimbabwe, 1991.

Comaroff, Jean. *Body of Power, Spirit of Resistance: The Culture and History of a South African People*. Chicago: University of Chicago Press, 1985.

Comaroff, Jean and John Comaroff. *Of revelation and revolution, Volume Two: The dialectics of modernity on a South African frontier*. Chicago: University of Chicago Press, 1997.

Cooper, Frederick. *Africa since 1940: The Past of the Present*. Cambridge: Cambridge University Press, 2002.

Cruz e Silva, Teresa. *Protestant Churches and the Formation of Political Consciousness in Southern Mozambique, 1930–1974*. Basel: P Schlettwein Publishing, 2001.

Cunningham, H. and J. Heyman. "Introduction: Mobilities and Enclosures at Borders." *Identities* 11, 2 (2004): 289–302.

Daneel, M. L. *Zionism and Faith-Healing in Rhodesia: Aspects of African Independent Churches*. The Hague: Mouton and Co, 1970.

Daneel, M. L. *Old and New in the Southern Shona Independent Churches, Volume I: Background and Rise of the Major Movements*. The Hague: Mouton & Co., 1971.

Fenner, Frank. "Smallpox: Emergence, Global Spread, and Eradication." *History and Philosophy of the Life Sciences* 15 (1993): 397–420.

Gelfand, Michael. *A Service to the Sick: A History of the Health Services for Africans in Southern Rhodesia, 1890–1953*. Gwelo: Mambo Press, 1976.

Greenough, Paul. "Intimidation, Coercion and Resistance in the Final Stages of the South Asian Smallpox Eradication Campaign, 1973–1975." *Social Science and Medicine* 41, 5 (1995): 633–45.

Herbert, Eugenia W. "Smallpox Inoculation in Africa." *Journal of African History* 16, 4 (1975): 539–559.

Isaacman, Allen and Isaacman, Barbara. *Mozambique: From Colonialism to Revolution, 1900–1982.* Boulder: Westview Press, 1983.

Johnson, Ryan and Amna Khalid. (Eds.) *Public Health in the British Empire: Intermediaries, Subordinates, and the Practice of Public Health, 1850–1960.* Routledge: New York, 2012.

Liesegang, Gerhard J. "Famines, Epidemics, Plagues and Long Periods of Warfare: Their Effects in Mozambique, 1700–1975." Paper presented at the Conference on Zimbabwean History: Progress and Development, University of Zimbabwe, 23–27 August 1982.

Mukonyora, Isabel. "Foundations for Democracy in Zimbabwe Evangelical Christianity." In *Evangelical Christianity and Democracy in Africa*, edited by Terence O. Ranger. 131–160. Oxford: Oxford University Press, 2008.

Muyambo, Clever. "Medical History of Mutare: A Case Study of the City's Health Services, 1960–1992." MA Thesis, Department of Economic History, University of Zimbabwe, March 1995.

Phillips, Howard. *Epidemics: The Story of South Africa's Five Most Lethal Human Diseases.* Athens, Ohio University Press, 2012.

Ranger, Terence. "The Early history of Independency in Rhodesia." In *Religion in Africa: proceedings of a seminar held in the Centre of African Studies*, University of Edinburgh, 10th–12th April, 1964.

Ranger, Terence. "Religious Movements and Politics in sub-Saharan Africa." *African Studies Review* 29, 2 (1986): 1–69.

Ranger, Terence. "Plagues of Beasts and Men; Prophetic Responses to Epidemics in Eastern and Southern Africa." In *Epidemics and Ideas: Essays in the Historical Perception of Pestilence*, edited by Terence Ranger and Paul Slack. 241–268. Cambridge: Cambridge University Press, 1992.

Ranger, Terence. "Taking on the Missionary's Task: African Spirituality and the Mission Churches of Manicaland in the 1930s." *Journal of Religion in Africa* 29, 2 (1999): 175–205.

Ranger, Terence. "Introduction." In *Evangelical Christianity and Democracy in Africa*, edited by Terence O. Ranger. 3–36. Oxford: Oxford University Press, 2006.

Ranger, Terence. "African Initiated Churches." *Transformation: An International Journal of Holistic Mission Studies* 24, 2 (2007): 65–71.

Ransford, O. *Bid the Sickness Cease: Disease in the History of Black Africa.* London: John Murray Publishers, 1983.

Schneider, William H. "The Long History of Smallpox Eradication: Lessons for Global Health in Africa." In *Global Health in Africa: Historical Perspectives on Disease*, edited by James L. A. Webb, JR. and Tamara Giles-Vernick. 25–41. Athens: Ohio University Press, 2013.

Sundkler, Bengt. *Bantu Prophets in South Africa*. London: International African Institute, 1961.

Vaughan, Megan. *Curing Their Ills: Colonial Power and African Illness*. Stanford: Stanford University Press, 1993.

Viljoen, Russell Stafford. "Disease. Doctors and De Beers Capitalists: Smallpox and Scandal in Colonial Kimberley (South Africa) during the Mineral Revolutions and British Imperialism, c. 1882–1883." In *Biomedicine as a Contested Site: Some Revelations in Imperial Contexts*, edited by Poonam Bala. 153–169. Lanham, MD: Lexington Books, 2009.

World Health Organization. Yaws, Fact Sheet no. 316. (February, 2014). http://www.who.int/mediacentre/factsheets/fs316/en/ (13 January 2015).

CHAPTER 7

Sexually Transmitted Diseases (STDs), the Border, and Public Health

It was in 1928 that Dr. Andrew Fleming, then the Medical Director for Zimbabwe, rebuked European settler claims, some even coming from health professionals, that the entire African population was rotten with syphilis.[1] This reflected the popular view among European settlers that all Africans, and in particular those from neighboring Mozambique, were diseased. Therefore, in addition to the well-documented concerns about African labor supply, settler fears of infection were a major impetus for the implementation of invasive public health measures among African men and women. However, most of these settler fears stemmed from misunderstandings of epidemiology by both the European settler public and health professionals, with race, ethnicity, the border, and paternalism playing a pivotal role in the European conception of the threat posed by sexually transmitted diseases (STDs).

As Europeans pursued science and medicine, "the final word in modern rationality," they were puzzled by the African reluctance to embrace the practices and values of Western biomedicine, which fanned fears of the potential of venereal diseases or STDs to "literally poison the body politic."[2] STDs were rarely fatal. Yet European settlers perceived them as

[1] NAZ S1173/220: Venereal Disease: Notes of a Conference held in the Committee Room, Municipal Offices, Bulawayo, on Saturday, October 6th, 1928.

[2] Philippa Levine, *Prostitution, Race and Politics: Policing Venereal Disease in the British Empire* (New York: Routledge, 2003), 9. In the colonial world, these diseases were referred to as venereal diseases, not sexually transmitted diseases.

F. Dube, *Public Health at the Border of Zimbabwe and Mozambique, 1890–1940*, African Histories and Modernities,
https://doi.org/10.1007/978-3-030-47535-2_7

a greater threat to their health. This was accompanied by baseless emphatic claims from medical authorities that tropical forms of STDs were "nastier and more potent" than European ones.[3] The truth, of course, was that these were the same diseases. It was just racism and colonialism at play. Thus, while control measures like examinations were implemented in the metropoles first, particularly among the urban poor women, what made the Zimbabwe-Mozambique border region unique was colonial rule. Even when other African colonies are considered, the peculiarities of a vicious type of colonialism, combined with border restrictions, made this unique. Also, while many studies have addressed various aspects of STDs in colonial Africa, none of these studies have focused on the implications of intercolonial borders in STD control.[4]

Studies have shown that from the late nineteenth well into the twentieth century, there was widespread belief in the prevalence of "innocent," meaning non-sexual spread of STDs, which increased fears and put pressure on colonial governments to identify, round up, and treat or, in the case of South Africa, jail those infected.[5] European settlers and some health professionals thought that they could contract venereal syphilis through articles of clothing, through sharing kitchen utensils, or by merely talking to a sufferer. This was a result of the confusion over diseases and pathogens, especially between non-venereal (yaws), known as *njovera* among the Shona, and venereal (syphilis) pathogens, which led to an overemphasis on the role of African sexuality in spreading STDs.[6] Settler fears were therefore based on erroneous understanding of STDs.

These embryonic and faulty understandings of STDs, particularly syphilis, and the fear they generated led to the implementation of some of the

[3] *Ibid.*

[4] See, for example, Guillaume Lachenal, "A Genealogy of Treatment as Prevention (TasP): Prevention, Therapy, and the Tensions of Public Health in African History," in *Global Health in Africa: Historical Perspectives on Disease*, ed. James L. A. Webb, JR. and Tamara Giles-Vernick (Athens: Ohio University Press, 2013), 79. See also Megan Vaughan, "Syphilis in Colonial East and Central Africa: The Social Construction of an Epidemic," in Epidemics and Ideas. Essays on the Historical Perception of Pestilence, ed. Terence Ranger and Paul Slack (Cambridge: Cambridge University Press, 1992), 269–302.

[5] Alan Jeeves, "Introduction: Histories of Reproductive Health and the Control of Sexually Transmitted Disease in Southern Africa: A Century of Controversy," *South African Historical Journal* 45 (2001): 2–3.

[6] Guillaume Lachenal, "A Genealogy of Treatment as Prevention (TasP), 79. See also Megan Vaughan, "Syphilis in Colonial East and Central Africa, 269–302.

most intrusive methods of public health such as restrictions on African mobility, medical "inspections" or "examinations," combined with pervasive condemnation of African peoples and their cultures. These settlers' views on the epidemiology of syphilis, as well as various moral standpoints on the nature of African societies, reflected their social construction of syphilis.[7]

Consequently, Africans' low compliance with colonial public health was based in part on that recognition that European understandings of disease were not necessarily sound as well as on the inefficacious public health policy toward STDs. Africans knew very well that syphilis was sexually transmitted. That was why many young African men thought contracting syphilis symbolized sexual potency and transition to manhood.

Regardless of whether European settler fears were grounded in truth or not, these perceptions informed and directed public health interventions and often led to the implementation of discriminatory public health policies. Investigations on the prevalence of venereal disease among Africans revealed that the infection rates were lower than what the lay settler population, and even some medical professionals, claimed. Yet Africans still suffered from the consequences of epidemiological misunderstandings and settler fears based on exaggerated and unfounded STD prevalence rates. Colonial officials compelled African migrants, both male and female, to undergo humiliating medical examinations, which interfered with African ideas of privacy and masculinity. To most European settlers, therefore, paternalism was supreme, with them treating Africans as children who could be compelled to undergo the invasive examinations.

This chapter therefore shows the centrality of the border in the evolution of colonial public health policy to colonial attempts to control STDs, known among the Shona of both Mozambique and Zimbabwe as *Siki*.[8] In particular, it focuses on venereal syphilis. *Siki*, denoting serious STDs, was likely derived from the English word sick, which might justify the belief in the region and in other parts of Africa that venereal syphilis and gonorrhea were first introduced by Europeans.[9] In fact, Africans associated STDs with the areas of European settlement, such as mining compounds, urban centers, and farms. This chapter shows how the border

[7] Vaughan, "Syphilis in Colonial East and Central Africa," 299.

[8] To this day, when some Zimbabweans are not feeling well, they prefer to say they are "ill," rather than "sick," because "sick" can be interpreted as suffering from an STD.

[9] Green, *Indigenous Theories of Contagious Disease*, 139.

simultaneously generated fears of diffusion of STDs from Mozambique, while it also hindered the implementation of effective regional public health policy in the border region, where cross-border movements were extensive. Labor migrants and other travelers, unlike cattle keepers whose mobility was curtailed by the border game and cattle fences, regularly slipped across the border. Mozambicans living in proximity to the border were more likely to go to Zimbabwe than elsewhere and therefore were likely to encounter Colonial Zimbabwean public health measures, such as medical examinations for STDs. The border was therefore a site of public health inspections, contributing to the resentment of public health monitoring.

As this chapter demonstrates, there was much division and debate between lay settlers and medical professionals, particularly in Zimbabwe, who were under pressure from this white public to adopt views and policies which they did not think were correct. While senior medical authorities often held different views based on empirical research and observation, they could not dismiss pressure from the settler population, who had the right to vote and control their own destiny. This suggests that whereas in African societies, healers enjoyed much status and influence, in the European settler community, the more progressive medical professionals advocated views which provoked considerable opposition from the European settler public.

STD Prevalence Among Africans and European Settler Fears

As discussed earlier, African mobility increased substantially during the colonial period as colonial states depended on African laborers. The spread of venereal syphilis to Zimbabwe, for instance, was associated with migrant laborers who migrated to the industrial centers of South Africa and brought back with them diseases of industrialization, such as venereal syphilis and tuberculosis.[10] These cross-border movements and the perceived high STD prevalence rates among Africans later fueled settler fears of infection. Other Europeans feared that African communities would be

[10] Gelfand, *A Service to the Sick*, 25, Vaughan, *Curing their Ills*, 39. See also Randall M. Packard, *White plague, Black Labor: Tuberculosis and the Political Economy of Health and Disease in South Africa* (Berkeley: University of California Press, 1989).

unable to reproduce themselves, biologically or socially, thus affecting labor supply.[11]

Soon after the establishment of colonial rule in Zimbabwe, some NCs from various parts of the colony, including those from the border districts of Mutare and Chipinge began to report on the incidence of STDs, particularly syphilis. In these reports there was much confusion between venereal syphilis and yaws. Most of the cases that were reported as venereal syphilis turned out to be yaws because the principal reason for its spread was that infected persons, during the secondary stage of the eruption, ate and drank out of the same dishes as those not infected, that the majority of the sufferers were children, and that in some villages nearly the entire population was affected.[12]

The lay sections of the white settler community in Zimbabwe often cited baseless and exaggerated rates of infection among Africans in order to foster their perception of Africans as reservoirs of disease. As early as 1898, the NC Mutare, T. B. Hulley, commented on what Europeans viewed as the reasons for what the settler community considered high prevalence of STDs among Africans. Writing on African customs, particularly the practice of polygamy and *Roora/Lobola* (bride price), Hulley claimed that African women had "absolutely no say in their own disposal, many being sold before they were born or even before their mothers were grown up."[13] According to Hulley, marriage among Africans was "a lottery and the course of true love has but a poor chance of running smoothly." He claimed incorrectly that, as a result, "adultery and immorality" was rife among Africans as "a woman's virtue goes no further than her market value." Yet Hulley was surprised that with the circumstances prevailing at that time, when an influx of white men who were "away from responsibility, and home ties and self respect forgotten for that time, that the [African] women [had] not become prostitutes to the whites."[14]

As a result of the rampant fears of STDs, based as they were on a faulty understanding of epidemiology, beginning in the early 1900s, there were increasing calls from the settler community for government action to deal with the so-called social evil.[15] Despite these calls, in 1903 there was still

[11] Vaughan, *Curing Their Ills*, 68.

[12] Gelfand, *A Service to the Sick*, 24–26.

[13] NAZ N9/1/1–4: Native Commissioners—Reports, Annual Report for Umtali, 1 April, 1898.

[14] *Ibid.*

[15] Gelfand, *A Service to the Sick*, 26.

no lock hospital in Zimbabwe to segregate and treat STD patients. However, by 1908 the Colonial Zimbabwean Government had initiated efforts to deal with the problem when the Medical Department issued anti-syphilitic medicines free to NCs, missionaries, police, and others in a position to treat patients.[16] Officials reported "markedly beneficial results," but then Medical Director Dr. Fleming considered the segregation of syphilitic patients impractical in the rural areas preferring, instead, to rely on the distribution of these remedies.[17] This strategy was one of the reasons why NCs later reported that these treatments were popular among Africans. As shown in Chap. 8, Africans preferred out-patient to in-patient treatment because the former gave them some degree of control over the healing process.

In Mozambique, the *Chefe* of Manica district expressed his astonishment as early as October 1904, at the "high number" of STDs which resulted in a police hunt for African prostitutes and their examination at Macequece hospital for two days.[18] Other European observers in Mozambique also cited high rates of STDs in the border region. Writing in 1907, Guillaume Vasse claimed that syphilis prevalence rates were high among the Africans of Manica (which included Macequece, Moribane, and Mossurize, among other districts).[19] As a result of these "high rates" of STDs among Africans, in 1917, the *Chefe* of Manica district called for a weekly inspection of "prostitutes."[20]

In Zimbabwe, with increasing concern over the spread of STDs to new mining areas, the Public Health Department warned in 1915 of "grave danger" if Africans suffering from STDs came in contact with Europeans and advocated legislating for the better supervision and control of African

[16] The treatments included the following: bluestone in the 1890s, composed of copper sulfate, which was rubbed into the sores with fat and later shown to be useless against syphilis; a mixture of potassium iodide, mercury, and arsenic in the early 1900s; arsenical preparations, Salvarsan and Novarsenobillon, which became widely accepted as a proven treatment against syphilis in the post-First World War period; and the anti-bacterial drug Penicillin in the post-Second World War period.

[17] Gelfand, *A Service to the Sick*, 26. It is questionable how beneficial these interventions were given the fact that the early anti-syphilis medicines were not effective.

[18] AHM, FCM, Secretaria Geral-Relatórios, Caixa 126, Pasta 2638, Circumscrição de Manica-Secção de Saúde, Relatório do Mez de Outobro de 1904.

[19] Guillaume Vasse, "The Mozambique Company's Territory II," *Journal of the Royal African Society* 6, no. 24 (1907): 385.

[20] AHM, FCM, Secretaria Geral-Relatórios, Caixa 126, Pasta 2649, Circumscrição de Manica-Relatório anual dos serviços de Saúde do hospital de Macequece, 1917.

women.[21] Consequently, public health officials examined African mine and farm workers at recruiting centers prior to their employment.

Countrywide, as the towns grew, so did public concern over the possibility of the spread of STDs in them. As a result, municipal councils pressured the central government to provide facilities for the periodic examination of African employees in their towns in addition to treating those infected. These efforts were spearheaded by the Municipality of Bulawayo beginning in October 1916, with the Municipality of Salisbury joining the efforts in 1917 because councilors felt it was absurd to "protect" the mines while leaving the big population centers "unprotected."[22] The government therefore invoked the Native Registration Ordinance, 1901, amended in 1918, which authorized it to establish regulations for the compulsory medical examination and vaccination of Africans applying for certificates of registration or during the period of their employment. This legislation was implemented by the end of 1919, with the commencement of examination of all Africans in employment in Salisbury and Bulawayo and the out-patient and in-patient treatment of all cases of disease diagnosed through these examinations.[23]

This development was also a culmination of the apparent increase in the incidence of STDs among Africans reported during and after the First World War. Reporting on Zimbabwean towns, Medical Director A. M. Fleming wrote that the prevalence of venereal diseases among Africans, both in employment and "casuals," was yearly becoming more serious.[24] He therefore urged the government to adopt measures for the detection, segregation, and treatment of these cases, warning that there was no system of any kind whatsoever for the isolation and treatment of STDs in any of the towns, "regardless of the fact that many of these affected natives may be in domestic service and expose innocent [white] persons to considerable risk."[25] According to Fleming, one of the reasons for the delay in erecting special wards for treating STDs stemmed from the lack of agreement on whether the cost was to be borne by the central government or the municipalities concerned.

[21] Vaughan, "Syphilis in Colonial East and Central Africa," 286–287.

[22] Gelfand, *A Service to the Sick*, 31.

[23] *Ibid.*, 33.

[24] NAZ, A3/12/6/1: Correspondence from A. M. Fleming, Medical Director, to the Secretary, Department of the Administrator, Southern Rhodesia, 17th June, 1919.

[25] *Ibid.*

As STD fears increased, so did the social construction of these diseases. Some medical officers argued that single African women were responsible for spreading STDs. For example, Fleming wrote in 1919 that the continuous spread of STDs was undoubtedly partly due to a certain class of African women, "mostly aliens from the north," who traveled from mine to mine, and between town locations, and who live on the proceeds of prostitution, or attach themselves to one African man for a time as his temporary wife.[26] He therefore considered it logical to attack what he regarded the root of the mischief and institute a system of examination and control of these women, but he acknowledged that this would probably entail special legislation.

These calls for special legislation to impose medical examinations on Africans were driven by what settlers believed to be a high prevalence of STDs among Africans, particularly those from Mozambique. In 1920 the NCs Mutare and Chipinge reported one death in each district resulting from STDs, but the NC Chipinge made the remark that his district was free from syphilis with the majority of the cases being contracted by Africans working outside the district.[27] Three years later, the NC Mutare claimed that after "extensive enquiries," it appeared that 600 Africans were suffering from STDs in his district, with about 450 of them suffering from syphilis and the rest from gonorrhea.[28] He decried the dearth of laws authorizing compulsory examination and treatment of "any one section of the community" and urged the government to take steps to provide hospital accommodation for Africans suffering from STDs. The NC asserted that the provision of separate hospital accommodation was important because STD patients who were being excluded from ordinary hospitals and unable to help themselves, were a "serious menace to public health, to say nothing of the suffering of the patients themselves."[29]

In that same year, the NC Chipinge reported two deaths from syphilis and noted that although there were no alarming figures, STDs had firmly

[26] NAZ, A3/12/6/1: Correspondence from A. M. Fleming, Medical Director, to the Secretary, Department of the Administrator, Southern Rhodesia, 17th June, 1919.

[27] NAZ, S2076: Native Commissioners-Reports, Report of the Native Commissioner, Melsetter District, for the year ended 31st December, 1920.

[28] NAZ, S235/501: District Reports-Native Commissioners, Report of the Native Commissioner, Umtali District, for the year ended 31st December, 1923.

[29] *Ibid.*

established themselves in the African population.[30] The NC also urged the government to take steps to eradicate these diseases. Thus beliefs about rampant widespread of STDs among Africans began to make their way into the settler public as were the calls for compulsory medical examination of Africans.

Even with the legislation put into force in 1919, the European public in Zimbabwe still felt that these efforts were not enough to deal with this "social evil." Hence, at a 1923 missionary conference, the delegates called for segregation, accompanied by the establishment of central lock hospitals.[31] They also demanded the building of accommodations in all towns for the temporary detention of STD and leprous patients waiting for hospital disposal, citing annual reports of NCs, who were concerned that African STD patients were not being admitted to government hospitals.

The year 1923 was also crucial for Zimbabwe because that was the year when the chartered British South Africa Company rule ended and white settlers adopted Responsible Government, with the power to elect a prime minister and members of the Legislative Council, as well as enjoying some degree of independence from Britain. Hence the following year witnessed the drafting of the Public Health Act (passed in 1925) with provisions for compulsory medical examination for and isolation of STD cases. With all these powers in their hands, it was not surprising that European settlers heightened their criticism of the government, calling for discriminatory public health measures against Africans.

In 1924 the NC Mutare was concerned about the increase in STD cases although he did not cite any statistics. He claimed that syphilis was on the increase and that "loose [African] women were the source of evil."[32] The NC was grateful for the Public Health Act, which would enable the compulsory examination of African women who frequented towns and mining camps. Mutare was said to be particularly vulnerable to STDs because apart from being a major eastern town, it was also close to Penhalonga, a mining town to the north, as well as Mozambique, long considered a hotbed of disease by Rhodesians. In that same year, the NC Chimanimani, south of Mutare, reported that he did not notice any increase in

[30] NAZ, S235/501: District Reports-Native Commissioners, Report of the Native Commissioner, Melsetter District, for the year ended 31st December, 1923.

[31] Gelfand, *A Service to the Sick*, 27.

[32] NAZ, S235/502: District Reports-Native Commissioners, Report of the Native Commissioner, Umtali District, for the year ended 31st December, 1924.

the incidence of STDs.[33] Yet reports from government medical officers, other NCs, and missionaries from various districts continued to show the high prevalence of STDs among Africans. Public health officials acknowledged that they did not have sufficient reliable statistics which might indicate whether or not the diseases were increasing among the African population.[34] The Medical Department thus began to take a less alarmist and more cautious approach, confronted by these glaring difficulties in measuring the incidence of STDs in the African population, and warned against overstating the incidence, which was the case elsewhere in Africa at this time, as "treatment became more popular as it became more effective."[35] However, many settlers believed that the disease was rampant and needed urgent attention.

In response, Fleming devised a medical scheme for treating STDs in Africans by requesting that the patients be "collected" and examined at a convenient center. In addition, starting in 1924 the central government paid missionaries £250 and furnished the necessary drugs for the treatment of syphilis.[36] Thus in the 1920s, the spread of STDs among Africans in both African reserves and on mines had been the subject of constant discussion on the part of the Native Department officials, missionaries, and the Legislative Council. However, before the passage of the Public Health Act in 1925, neither the government nor local authorities had sufficient powers to deal with what public health officials considered a "pressing and outstanding menace to the public health and the future child life of the native population."[37] Hence, Chapter III of the Public Health Act dealt entirely with STDs, which, according to officials, was "a public health question of primary importance" in Zimbabwe, "more especially as it affect[ed] the native population."[38]

The decades that followed the proclamation of the Public Health Act witnessed the adoption of vigorous and sometimes racist measures to arrest the "menace" of STDs. These measures included medical examinations of African men and women in towns and mining centers. African

[33] NAZ, S235/502: District Reports-Native Commissioners, Report of the Native Commissioner, Melsetter sub-District, for the year ended 31st December, 1924.

[34] NAZ, S2419: Report on the Public Health for the Year 1924, Southern Rhodesia.

[35] Vaughan, "Syphilis in Colonial East and Central Africa," 287.

[36] Gelfand, *A Service to the Sick*, 27.

[37] NAZ, A3/12/25 Health and Medical Services: Public Health Act, September 17, 1920–February 18, 1925.

[38] *Ibid.*

men, including those from neighboring colonies, such as Mozambique, Zambia, and Malawi, were examined for STDs before they could be employed in urban and mining centers. African women increasingly came to be viewed by colonial officials as the source of evil as they assumed that independent African women were prostitutes, spreading gonorrhea and syphilis in towns and mines. Yet, as Lawrence Vambe notes, for Europeans, particularly colonial officials, this "prostitution" by African women was "a blessing in disguise, for it safeguarded the chastity of white womanhood from the lust of their male native servants."[39] He argues that between the First and Second World Wars, professional prostitutes in Harare, for example, appeared to enjoy some sort of official recognition because they acquired accommodation as easily as legitimately employed male workers.

Nonetheless, colonial officials examined women entering urban and mining areas for STDs.[40] For instance, from March to December 1925, public health officials examined 6136 Africans in Bulawayo and treated 30 cases of syphilis and 8 of gonorrhea.[41] During the same year, public health officials examined 10,444 Africans and treated 74 cases of syphilis and 13 of gonorrhea. Pressured by the European public, from 1926, the Medical Department implemented what it called a "crusade" against STDs, through the setting up of clinics and nudging local authorities in urban areas to assume more responsibility for treatments and control.[42]

These inspections were also dictated by the interests of capital, for they ascertained a man's suitability for labor. Industry wanted to keep to an absolute minimum the cost of maintaining a healthy labor force. "Inspections" had to fulfill this duty of keeping reservoirs of infection from reaching mining compounds. Thus, in addition to STD examinations, African men seeking employment also had to undergo medical examinations for tuberculosis, scabies, leprosy, and ringworm.

However, concern over STDs continued to grow. The NC Chipinge expressed this in 1926. Considering that American Board missionaries had been working in the district continuously for 30 years, he felt disappointed

[39] Lawrence Vambe, *From Rhodesia to Zimbabwe* (Pittsburgh: University of Pittsburgh Press, 1976), 185.

[40] Philippa Levine notes that this targeting of women did not start in the colonies, but in Britain itself, where women campaigners opposed the double standard: "only women were responsible for disease transmission and thus liable to legal and medical surveillance." See Levine, *Prostitution, Race and Politics*, 2.

[41] Gelfand, *A Service to the Sick*, 33–34.

[42] Vaughan, "Syphilis in Colonial East and Central Africa," 287.

at what he considered the "small progress" made by Africans as a whole in the district.[43] To account for the perceived increase in the incidence of STDs, the NC argued that, with the exception of the comparatively small African communities that clustered around the European-controlled mission stations of Mt. Selinda and Chikore, there was nowhere among the adult generation "any recognition of the need for improvement." He added that polygamy, which he considered to be the strongest of all inhibitions against change, was the general practice and claimed that even the chiefs were never progressive. On the contrary, the NC said that these chiefs were backward and that the drinking of beer often continued "till far into the night with intermittent dancing while sexual irregularities" were "winked at by the older people," who themselves had become unfit to enforce restraint.[44] These were the practices that settlers considered to be behind the perceived high incidence of STDs.

Yet, while European settlers thought that all Africans were infected with STDs, surveys of the prevalence of these diseases among Africans showed that European settler fears were exaggerated. In 1928 the Medical Director for Zimbabwe, Dr. A. M. Fleming, chided settlers, saying,

> On this subject, a good deal of nonsense has been talked, and one is constantly confronted with loose statements on the prevalence of venereal disease among the native races; in fact, it is not uncommon thus to hear a responsible person, who should know better, give it as their considered opinion that up to 80 per cent or 90 per cent of the native population are syphilitic, or to hear the more careless expression "*the whole lot of them are rotten with syphilis.*"[45]

It was alarming that even "responsible person[s]," presumably physicians, also discarded known facts and joined in the chorus of unfounded claims of STD incidence that prevailed within the lay European settler population. The perception was the same in other parts of colonial Africa. In Uganda, for instance, an established authority, Colonel Lambkin of the Royal Army Medical Corps, estimated that 80 percent of the African population was infected with syphilis, resulting in infant mortality rates of

[43] NAZ S235/504 Native Commissioners-Reports, Report of the Native Commissioner for Melsetter District, for the Year ending 31st December, 1926.

[44] *Ibid.*

[45] NAZ S1173/220: Venereal Disease: Notes of a Conference held in the Committee Room, Municipal Offices, Bulawayo, on Saturday, October 6th, 1928. Emphasis added.

50–60 percent, which, according to him, threatened the survival of the "race."[46] In Zimbabwe, however, Fleming argued that STD prevalence rates among Africans were much lower than commonly assumed. For example, in 1928 Fleming noted that of the 110,000 African male adults examined for STDs, the incidence of syphilis (in clinical form) among them was approximately 2–3 percent or to 20–30 per thousand, "not an excessive or alarming figure and indeed one which compares favourably with similar returns from our own [British] army and navy."[47]

However, despite these assurances from the medical community, settlers continued to claim that STDs were rampant among Africans and blamed African customs and lifestyle for the prevalence. In 1929, Mary W. Waters, the Organizing Instructress in the Native Education Department, urged settlers to act on what she considered "vices" among Africans, arguing "Are we to leave them [Africans] with these vices. Are we to shut our eyes to people who live in a state of terror, darkness, poverty and filth; *with the most degraded sexual practices, and consequently with disease and suffering rife among them*?"[48] Little wonder European settlers perceived Africans as a reservoir of disease. Some sections of the European community, particularly lay settlers, considered *all* Africans to be syphilitic owing to their way of life, leading to calls for more government intervention. Much of this denigration of African customs, however, came from misunderstanding and lack of will to learn African ways.

The administration therefore made an effort to combat STDs wherever they were believed to be prevalent. On mines, infected African mineworkers were sent to one of the four STD clinics available by 1929, but the

[46] Vaughan, "Syphilis in Colonial East and Central Africa," 269.

[47] NAZ, S1173/220: Venereal Disease: Notes of a Conference held in the Committee Room, Municipal Offices, Bulawayo, on Saturday, October 6th, 1928. This total of 110,000 included Africans residing in urban areas, African prisoners in goals, members of the Native Police Force, African patients under treatment in government hospitals, and Africans who were looking for work on mines and railways. All these were under direct European control and subject to medical examination and treatment when sick. Fleming was referring to the British Army and Navy, noting that the incidence of venereal disease in the navy for the year 1926 was 7 percent. This meant that of the total naval population of about 90,000 men, 6453 of them were suffering from venereal disease.

[48] NAZ, S1173/337–338: Address on the work among Native women and girls in Southern Rhodesia given to the members of the welfare society and others in Bulawayo, March 13th, 1929, by Mary W. Waters, Organizing Instructress, Native Education Department, Rhodesia.

mine was responsible for their fees.[49] Three of these clinics were entirely run by the municipalities of Harare, Bulawayo, and Mutare, albeit with substantial assistance from the central government. In addition, there were other clinics at mission stations. As an expression of the great fear of STDs in the settler community and the need for more action, in 1931 Mr. Guy Taylor, Chief Clerk in the Health Department, indicated that the main objective of rural hospitals in Zimbabwe was to curtail the spread of STDs.[50]

It was the same story in Mozambique involving the condemnation of African cultural practices as major contributors to the prevalence of STDs. A 1929 health services report asserted that alcoholism and STDs among Africans posed a grave threat to the public. The report claimed the Africans lacked notions of hygiene and that because Africans lived in communities where prostitution abounded, they were often fatal victims of STDs.[51] The report recommended the development of measures to prevent the spread of STDs. Included among these measures were attempts to curb prostitution.[52]

Perceptions of Africans as reservoirs of disease persisted, with exaggerated STD prevalence rates culminating in the assumption that "the whole lot of them are rotten with syphilis." In Zimbabwe, the American Board Mission Hospital at Mt. Selinda reported having treated 89 cases of syphilis and yaws in 1930 and 208 cases in 1931, with STDs being the second "great offender" among Africans after malaria.[53] For the missionaries, venereal syphilis justified their work as they tied what they considered inherent sinfulness of traditional African society to disease, citing polygyny in particular and rejected theories that blamed Christianity for the "deculturation" of Africans, resulting in the spread of syphilis. [54]

It was during this period, the 1930s, that in some parts of Central Africa, such as Zambia and Malawi, there was increasing concern over the ability of rural populations to reproduce themselves and especially in those

[49] Gelfand, A Service to the Sick, 27–29.

[50] *Ibid.*, 29.

[51] AHM, FCM, Secretaria Geral-Relatórios, Caixa 128, Pasta 2678, Relatório da Direcção dos Serviços de Saúde-Assistência Sanitaria ao Indigena, 1929, 3.

[52] *Ibid.*

[53] NAZ, S2014/6/2: American Board Mission, 1925–1947, Report of Medical work—Mount Selinda Mission, 1931 and 1932.

[54] Vaughan, "Healing and Curing Issues," 135–136 and Vaughan, "Syphilis in Colonial East and Central Africa," 270.

supplying migrant labor.[55] Yet, while much of the focus was on syphilis, gonorrhea, which typically causes scarring of the fallopian tubes, resulting in sterility, was more likely the cause of infertility in women.[56]

The 1930s thus witnessed continued demands to extend medical examinations to more Africans and concerns about cross-border movements, especially in border towns such as Mutare. In 1933 the Medical Officer for Mutare, Oswald E. Jackson, pressed for the compulsory medical examination of Africans, citing the "proximity of the Portuguese Border" in relation to Mutare, "as a large number of P.E.A. [Portuguese East Africa/Mozambique] natives obtain work here [in Mutare]."[57] He added that it was not likely that these migrants could obtain medical assistance in Mozambique as easily as in Zimbabwe. Jackson's claim suggests that the European settlers' fear of Africans, and migrants from Mozambique in particular, as reservoirs of disease was heightened by the proximity to the Mozambican border and how the border affected settler imagination by stirring up fear of an unfamiliar "other" territory, which in this case was not far away.

Although Jackson argued that the danger of an African servant infecting a member of a European household was remote, he stressed, there "is a very decided fear of infection in the [European] public mind."[58] This fear led to calls for compulsory examination of Africans. As demonstrated already, a system to force *all employed* Africans in urban areas to undergo medical examination for STDs was already in place by 1933, but the Mutare Town Council wanted this system to be extended to all Africans *seeking work*. One settler, Mr. Malcom, told then the Medical Director R. A. Askins that Mutare's European population feared that Africans seeking work would infect the European population with STDs.[59] However, Askins pushed back on these claims, arguing that it was not clear upon what grounds these fears were based, but it might be stated that STDs

[55] Vaughan, "Syphilis in Colonial East and Central Africa," 288.

[56] Tuck, "Kabaka Mutesa and Venereal Disease," 313, 325.

[57] NAZ S246/343: Umtali, Natives-Medical Examination, 1937–48, Correspondence from Umtali Medical Director, Oswald E. Jackson to the Secretary, Department of the Colonial Secretary, Southern Rhodesia, 5th May, 1933.

[58] *Ibid.*

[59] NAZ S246/343: Umtali, Natives-Medical Examination, 1937–48, Correspondence from the Medical Director, Southern Rhodesia to The Secretary, Department of the Colonial Secretary, Southern Rhodesia, 5th May, 1933.

were not spread from one person to another in this manner and that the Mutare Town Council had overstated the danger of infection.[60]

Another example of this fear of infections was shown by the European settler, Colonel H. A. Stewart, who castigated the government's "neglect" of STDs. Stewart's African employee had been diagnosed with STDs. He wrote, angrily in 1938,

> I ... feel most strongly that the Government Medical Authorities of Southern Rhodesia are guilty of culpable negligence in allowing a system to exist in this country whereby the white population, and more especially the women and children are exposed to the risk of infection from this terrible disease .... Therefor[e] it stands to reason some means should exist whereby a native suffering from venereal [disease] was compelled by law to state the fact or to produce some document showing the disease he was suffering from and this should not necessarily be confined to venereal [disease] as there are other diseases such as tuberculosis which though not so horrible may be even more deadly.[61]

To emphasize his point, Stewart wrote about his experience in the British Army where, he claimed, a medical history sheet was kept for every Regular Soldier under Commissioned rank. He said it was a crime, under the Army Act, for "ANY" soldier, regardless of rank, to conceal the fact that he was suffering from an STD. Yet a system which was devised for the health and general well-being of the British Regular Army, continued Stewart, "*composed as it is of well educated, cultured white men is apparently considered by the Government Officials of Southern Rhodesia as degrading to a black African native who less than a century ago was in the most literal sense a savage and today is very little, if any, better.*"[62] Just like in other British territories, the military authorities defended the moral reputation of their soldiers and blamed the spread of sexually transmitted diseases directly on African prostitutes. Yet it was telling that while the civil authorities condemned the coercive methods used by the military to control the spread

[60] *Ibid.*

[61] NAZ, S482/534/39: Natives-Medical Examination, 1937–48, Correspondence from Colonel H. A. Stewart to the Minister of Native Affairs for Southern Rhodesia, 11th April 1938.

[62] *Ibid.* Emphasis added.

of these diseases, particularly the forced examination of European women,[63] they advocated the very same methods for African women.

In addition, such racist language, as quoted above, was commonly used in comments on non-whites. While investigating the sources of STDs in 1947, one of the Public Health Department committee members, Lt. Col. Appleby claimed, "Coloured females particularly are responsible for a good proportion of V.D. [venereal disease] of Europeans and therefore a number of the names reported to local health authorities would be of persons of these races."[64] Every effort therefore had to be devoted to stopping infection from reaching Europeans. Colonel Stewart, for instance, in his letter to the Minister of Native Affairs clearly stated,

> I understand from the press that this Government [Rhodesia] is about to bring in legislation to encourage and financially assist the immigration of a good class of white settler. May I ask, Sir, with every respect whether these immigrants are going to be warned that its Government takes no steps whatsoever to safeguard them against the greatest scourge known to man. Under existing regulations all immigrants have, apparently, to satisfy the Immigration Officers that they are free from tuberculosis yet with amazing inconsistency the Medical Authorities of Southern Rhodesia not only permit, but by their passive, non-committal attitude actually encourages a far worse and more horrible disease to stalk unchecked through the land. And this at a time when all great nations of the world are doing their utmost to improve the standard of health of their peoples and particularly of the young generation.[65]

Attracting a "good class of white settler" was of paramount importance in Zimbabwe, which faced stiff competition from South Africa, Kenya, and some British dominions, such as Australia, New Zealand, and Canada. For European settlers, populating the colony with white settlers was the basis of survival given that the African population always far outnumbered the white population. Many white settlers believed that there was a need for

[63] Vaughan, "Healing and Curing Issues," 145.

[64] NAZ, S2014/3/10: Plague, 1937 February 5th–1947 April 30th, Notes of a meeting to discuss the tracing and investigation of infection of venereal disease held in the Public Health Department on 5th November 1947. Colored people were those of mixed races, particularly between white and black.

[65] NAZ, S482/534/39: Natives-Medical Examination, 1937–48, Correspondence from Colonel H. A. Stewart to the Minister of Native Affairs for Southern Rhodesia, 11th April 1938.

more white settlers to occupy the land, "develop" it, and defend it from the more numerous Africans. Under such conditions, it is not surprising that the government was compelled by settler arguments to implement tough public health laws. In any case, with the advent of Responsible Government in Zimbabwe in 1923, power lay in the white settlers, the only ones who had the right to vote for government officials. Protection of white settler privilege and health was central to the survival of settler colonies. As Colonel Stewart lamented, "The present state of affairs in regard to *venereal disease among the native population and the terrible danger of its infection to the white people is a disgrace to this Government and their Medical Authorities.*"[66]

While Stewart vigorously advocated compulsory medical examination of Africans for STDs, then Medical Director, Andrew Paton Martin, responded by saying that Stewart's complaint reflected "the old story of compulsion, but always compulsion for somebody else … but as you know, compulsion has been abandoned long ago by most public health departments who ever attempted to deal with this condition."[67] Martin wondered how Colonel Stewart would react if he were asked to carry about a medical history sheet and submit to medical examination whenever somebody else thought he ought to do so. Stewart's premise, however, was that Africans were "savages" and thus could be compelled to undergo invasive public health measures because they were not at par with "well educated, cultured white" people. Nevertheless, Martin did not succeed in reducing racist influence on public health. If anything, it was largely this pressure from the settler community that led to the formulation of public health policy, just as any nation responds to the pleas of its citizens.

Most of the European settlers therefore expressed a lack of understanding of the epidemiology of STDs. Medical Director R. A. Askins had once lamented, the "lay people have an exaggerated dread of venereal disease," adding that many thought that all Africans had it and that one could become infected by simply talking to a sufferer.[68] However, this expression of ignorance might have been a convenient way through which these lay Europeans tried to absolve themselves of immoral activities, such as

[66] *Ibid.* Emphasis added.

[67] NAZ S482/534/39: Natives-Medical Examination, 1937–48, Letter from Andrew Paton Martin, Medical Director, to the Prime Minister, Southern Rhodesia, 23rd April, 1938.

[68] NAZ S1173/332–334, Letter from the Medical Director, Southern Rhodesia, R. A. Askins to The Secretary, Department of Internal Affairs, Southern Rhodesia, 31st October, 1933.

prostitution. Fears of infection and the need to find scapegoats therefore led European settlers to blame Africans for STDs as Askins indicated in 1939,

> The [white] Public's attitude towards this examination [for venereal syphilis] is ... an ill-informed one, but is based on the very genuine fear that exists against exposure to infection and the contraction of these diseases. But this fear is not well-founded and the dangers of the risk of infection are grossly exaggerated. All these awful tales of the contraction of infection from closet-seats, towels, drinking cups, are just so much moonshine and for the most part are the inventions of persons who are driven to all sorts of expedients to explain the origin of the venereal disease from which they are suffering. These stories are the common currency of the doctor's consulting room and medical men have long learned to maintain discreet silence in the face of these voluble explanations.[69]

As Askins alluded, some of these explanations could have been deliberate distortions in order to shift the blame to Africans.

As mentioned earlier, part of the problem was the inability to distinguish venereal syphilis from non-venereal syphilis or framboesia (yaws). According to Fleming, most of the claims of high rates of infection in rural areas were estimates which were difficult to make because STDs, particularly syphilis, had symptoms similar to those of leprosy and framboesia, both of which were "common" among Africans. Thus, according to Fleming, a certain proportion of cases reported by various treatment centers countrywide as STDs were actually framboesia or yaws. He indicated that framboesia was a disease of African villages which was exceedingly prevalent in tropical and sub-tropical parts of Africa such as Kenya, Tanzania (Tanganyika), the Democratic Republic of Congo (Belgian Congo), Congo-Brazzaville, and in certain areas of Zimbabwe. Distinguishing between framboesia and syphilis was difficult because both diseases had similar primary, secondary, and tertiary stages.[70] Hence it was difficult for social workers and public health authorities to give correct estimates as regards the incidence of STDs, particularly among Africans in rural areas.

[69] NAZ S482/534/39: Natives-Medical Examination, 1937–48, Letter from the Medical Director, Southern Rhodesia, to the Minister of Internal Affairs, Southern Rhodesia, 11th January, 1939.

[70] *Ibid.*

Similar associations of Africans with STDs were also made in Mozambique as hospitals recorded several cases of STDs among Africans. The Mozambique Company's hospital records suggest that syphilis was the most prevalent of all STDs.[71] The Manica district, for example, registered 17 cases of syphilis in 1917, 5 cases in 1935, 33 cases in 1939, and 47 cases in 1940, whereas Mossurize district registered 2 cases in 1939 and 10 cases in 1940. As for other STDs, Manica district registered 20 cases in 1935, 21 cases in 1939, and 22 cases in 1940 while Mossurize district registered 3 cases in 1939 and 1 case in 1940.[72] Owing to the fact that the Manica district had larger urban centers than Mossurize, it was bound to have more STD cases. Overall, the data generated by public health officials did not substantiate the notion of widespread incidence of venereal disease among Africans.

In fact, the incidence of STDs was small. Even when considering these annual infection rates against the total African population under the Mozambique Company government in 1909, which was 237,941, one finds that the infection rates were negligible.[73] These infection rates did not warrant alarm even when considering the population of one district alone. For instance, the total African population of Mossurize district was estimated at 25,305 in 1935, at 35,037 in 1936, at 36,712 in 1937, and at 38,222 by 1938.[74]

Furthermore, to back up their claims of high STD prevalence among Africans, European settlers claimed that the source of STDs was "primarily in the native districts, and spreading from there to the centres of European occupation and was becoming a menace to the white population."[75] Yet inquiries made by public health officials to determine the prevalence of syphilis continuously demonstrated that STDs were spreading *from* the towns and centers of European settlement toward and not from African districts because urban areas had a higher percentage of STD incidence

[71] AHM, FCM, Secretaria Geral-Relatórios, Caixa 119, Pasta 2294, Direcção dos Serviços de Saúde, 1936, 1937, 1938, 1939, and 1940.

[72] *Ibid.*

[73] AHM, FCM, Secretaria Geral-Relatórios, Recenciamento da População da Europea, e Indigena, Territorio de Manica e Sofala, 24th March 1909, Box no. 193, File no. 636.

[74] AHM, FCM, Secretaria Geral-Relatórios, Report of the District of Mossurize for the Year 1935, 1936, 1937 and 1938, box no. 266.

[75] NAZ, S1173/220: Venereal Disease: Notes of a Conference held in the Committee Room, Municipal Offices, Bulawayo, on Saturday, October 6th, 1928.

than the rural areas.[76] Due to this data, in Zimbabwe, Fleming finally realized that the incidence of STDs among Africans in towns and mining centers was not so much influenced by contact with Europeans as by the working and living conditions in towns. As he pointed out, most of the unskilled labor was undertaken by male adult Africans who, while in employment, were divorced from family life and among whom cohabitation and promiscuity with African women was accordingly common.[77] He noted that in 1926 there were 110,041 African males employed in urban and mining areas while only 2908 African females resided in these same areas. The problem was that the largest number of these employed males came from neighboring colonies as temporary immigrants seeking work, without their wives and families.[78] Fleming added that of these "3,000 African females distributed among 110,000 male Africans" in urban and mining centers, the majority of them were prostitutes and this accounted for the increasing incidence of STDs in Zimbabwe.

As Fleming noted, the STD issue was primarily a social and economic problem which could have been addressed by ameliorating the social conditions of migrant African workers in urban and mining centers through the provision of decent family units and "family wages," not "bachelor wages." It was not entirely a medical problem. This mirrored what had been experienced in South Africa. As elsewhere in colonial Africa, despite calls to identify, round up, and treat or jail those infected, officials realized that mass treatment was difficult or impossible because of the costs involved, the prolonged treatment regimens with less effective drugs available before antibiotics, and the simple medical infrastructure, particularly in the rural areas.[79] By the 1930s, as many public health officials recognized that labor migration was a factor in the transmission of these and other infectious diseases, some physicians acknowledged as well that rampant poverty in both black rural and urban areas increased African susceptibility to these diseases.

Yet, even as the South African Department of Public Health realized the role of poverty in the spread of epidemic infectious disease, there was a conspicuous disconnect between the "emerging social explanation of disease" and distinct public health methods formulated to deal with them.

[76] *Ibid.*

[77] *Ibid.*

[78] *Ibid.*

[79] Jeeves, "Introduction: Histories of Reproductive Health," 3.

Hence, the public health methods of the 1930s and 1940s depended more on curative medicine and rudimentary health education than on ameliorating the underlying social and economic conditions such as housing, welfare, environmental sanitation, and anti-poverty programs.[80]

It was the same in Kenya, where bachelor housing, built on the understanding that migrant laborers temporarily accommodated by employers would not live with their spouses and children, had been provided until the 1940s.[81] Here STD regulations came later with the 1921 and 1928 ordinances, listing venereal diseases as notifiable diseases and authorizing the Medical Officer of Health to remove an infected person to a hospital for treatment and to trace all contacts for examination and treatment if necessary.[82] This was accompanied by the rounding off of defaulters.[83] Among the challenges encountered was that, as the Public Health Department realized, STD patients actually represented a very small percentage of the perceived real prevalence of infection among Africans.

Public health officials also became aware of the fundamental factors that complicated STD control efforts, such as African mobility, great distances to hospitals, as well as bachelor housing.[84] To solve these problems the public health officials recommended, among other things, the establishment of sub-clinics and the provision of a traveling dispensary to visit distant districts regularly and a public campaign to educate victims on the need for sustained treatment even after the disappearance of symptoms. However, none of these suggestions were put into effect due to lack of funds and personnel. What officials considered the most effective preventive method was the control of the "influx of unemployed and unemployable African men and women" into towns, which led to the promulgation of the venereal diseases regulations of September 1944, empowering the police to pick up any African males and females and hand them over for medical examination to control prostitution in Nairobi.[85] Yet it was clear that the ultimate causation of prostitution was economic and social, stemming from the lack of family housing units and family wages in the urban areas. However, all this required higher wages, which employers, eager to minimize costs and maximize profits, would not agree to. As a result,

[80] *Ibid.*, 4.
[81] Achola, "The Public Health Ordinance Policy," p. 117.
[82] *Ibid.*
[83] *Ibid.*
[84] *Ibid.*, 124–125.
[85] *Ibid.*, 125.

colonial officials placed more emphasis on African "ignorance" as the cause of the perceived high prevalence of STDs and sought to educate Africans on these and "all other major enemies of public health," through traveling lecture clinics.[86]

Concern over STDs increased even further during the Second World War. In much of Central and Eastern Africa, including Mozambique and Zimbabwe, there was an increase in the reported incidence of STDs, especially syphilis and gonorrhea. This was mostly attributed to huge recruitment of large numbers of African men into the army and their mobility associated with the war effort.[87]

However, surveys on the prevalence of STDs among Africans continued to show that the numbers of those infected were small. In 1949, an STD survey in Zimbabwe "found the position not as serious as was thought" because the overall incidence of STDs was about 6 percent among 22,923 industrial workers, 3.6 percent among the 1653 men of the armed forces and police, and 1.6 percent among 121,045 other workers who were periodically examined.[88] Although officials attributed these low incidence rates to the government's anti-syphilitic program initiated in mid-1920s, these figures probably reflected what the *real* infection rates had been all along.

That the number of Africans infected with STDs was small was also shown in the following reports from the border district of Chipinge. In 1956 the NC Chipinge reported that 135 patients were treated for STDs at Biriwiri Government Clinic in the area bordering the Moribane district of Mozambique, representing "an increase on previous figures." The NC attributed this increase in cases to a "large road camp" that was operating in the vicinity. Further west, at Nyanyadzi Clinic, which served Marange Reserve, the Buhera-Save area as well as Chipinge District, the NC reported that 59 STD patients were treated, noting, however, that these patients "often decamp after the initial injection and are often rounded up as often as possible." He also reported that the orderly in charge was astute in "collecting" the wives of sufferers and examining them.[89] However, the numbers involved were small.

[86] *Ibid.*, 126.

[87] Vaughan, "Syphilis in Colonial East and Central Africa," 290.

[88] Gelfand, *A Service to the Sick*, 33.

[89] NAZ, S2827/2/2/4: Annual Report for the year ended 31st December, 1956, NC, Melsetter.

Failure to finish the full and lengthy course of syphilis treatment was common among African patients in the pre-penicillin era. Colonial officials reported that many African STD sufferers sought treatment, particularly for the first phase, after which they disappeared. However, this quest for treatment, culturally, put African patients into a dilemma, just as it exposed the contradictions inherent in Western medicine. If Africans presented themselves for treatment, as they did, Europeans were bewildered and felt their perceived superiority reinforced, with this African lack of "shame" sometimes interpreted as evidence of the illogical and perilous nature of Africans' sexuality.[90] Yet if Africans did not present themselves for treatment, colonial officials still condemned them. In fact, this was a classic example of Africans experimenting with and selectively adopting some aspects of Western biomedicine.

However, failure to finish the course of treatment only increased European fears about relapses and the potential for infection. Thus although STDs had been in decline since the 1860s, they still drew public and medical attention through their close connection to morality.[91] Part of this moral issue was the settlers' attempts to find ways of accounting for the origins of their STDs outside sexual contact, contributing to these unfounded theories of transmission, such as contracting venereal disease by simply talking to a sufferer. Colonial Zimbabwean Secretary for Health M. H. Webster deplored these erroneous settler views of STDs, which some professionals also embraced. He recalled in 1972,

> There was always then, as always, a curious pre-occupation with venereal disease. This was reflected in the prominence given to venereal diseases and the control thereof in the Public Health Act which was introduced in 1924 and promulgated in 1925. The superstitious awe with which the general [white] public views venereal disease is possibly understandable in view of the scandalous connotations of these conditions, but it is hard to see why a learned profession should consistently exaggerate the public health importance of syphilis and gonorrhea.[92]

[90] Vaughan, "Healing and Curing Issues," 150. For a more detailed discussion on the popularity of STD treatments, see Gelfand, *A Service to the Sick*, 24, Vaughan, "Syphilis in Colonial East and Central Africa," 286.

[91] Levine, *Prostitution, Race, and Politics*, 5.

[92] M. H. Webster, "A Review of the Development of the Health Services of Rhodesia from 1923 to the Present Day, Part I, the 1920s." *The Central African Journal of Medicine* 18, no. 12 (December, 1972): 246.

Thus, according to Webster, while the layman's misunderstanding of the transmission of STDs might have been genuine, that of learned professionals was inexcusable. Perhaps it was a question of the disjuncture between the "reasonableness and rationality" of the Medical Department concerning intervention and the "language of medicine," which emphatically warned of contagion from the African "reservoirs" of disease, fanning even more fears within the settler community.[93]

Africans became convenient scapegoats for settler misunderstanding of the epidemiology of STDs. Yet these Africans knew that venereal syphilis was a sexually transmitted disease and thought of it as having a primarily moral cause, often associated with prostitution and having extra-marital affairs, as some think now about HIV/AIDS. Africans also knew that syphilis, for instance, was a disease of cities and compounds on farms and mines. The name *Siki* itself, as derivation from English, suggests that Africans associated this disease more broadly with colonialism and the intrusion of Europeans than with precolonial African society. Thus, while colonial officials argued that prostitution was responsible for the spread of STDs, what they considered "prostitution" was then a new kind of sexual relationship which was associated with urban and compound life on European settler farms and mines. This "prostitution" was associated with colonial labor demands and wage employment which contributed to extensive labor migration.[94]

The "Efficacy" of Medical Examinations

In Zimbabwe, after the promulgation of the Public Health Act, the government secured all the powers needed to enforce medical examinations for STDs among Africans as a public health measure. This Act represented an extension of a system of medical exams which had started on the mines. Hence, women entering mining and urban centers and men seeking employment were examined for STDs. But what was the purpose and impact of these racially motivated medical exams? This is a crucial question because European settlers thought they would be protected from the so-called infective Africans by implementing compulsory medical examinations.

[93] Vaughan, "Syphilis in Colonial East and Central Africa," 287–288.

[94] For more on prostitution and STDs on Rhodesian mine compounds, see Van Onselen, *Chibaro*.

In order to finance these medical examinations, municipalities and local authorities demanded half of the town pass tax so they could place more Africans under medical examination. However, the Medical Director argued that in making this proposal, both central and local governments appeared to have attributed more significance to the public health merits of a medical exam than "present methods seem to warrant."[95] The main reason for his doubts was that this so-called medical examination was carried out by laymen, usually sanitary inspectors, and consisted merely of cursory inspection of Africans under circumstances not conducive to any more detailed examination even if this were desired. He argued that this type of medical examination was ineffective because the visible and "grosser" signs of infection were ephemeral in duration and disappeared long before the end of the infectious stage. For this reason, a small percentage of people suffering from STDs in a communicable form were detected by the medical exam. As a result, a large number of people who did not show external signs of the disease but who were nevertheless infected, and frequently highly infectious, were not detected at all.[96] The Public Health Department was aware of the limitations of this method of examination but held on to the belief that a small gain in the fight against STDs was better than none at all.

Furthermore, public health officials argued that another flaw of this type of examination and "other more trustworthy methods" was that the results obtained were only true for the actual time of examination. Thus, a person who was reasonably and justly certified to be free of STDs at the time of examination could an hour or two afterward contract the disease and become capable of transmitting. Yet the European public, despite all these warnings, continued to cling to the idea that medical examinations alone had some protective value which extended over indefinite periods of months. They believed that a recently examined person found to be uninfected could not possibly be suffering from the disease. These were, according to public health authorities, dangerous beliefs which led to an unjustifiable sense of security.[97]

[95] NAZ, S482/534/39: Natives-Medical Examination, 1937–48, Letter from the Medical Director, Southern Rhodesia, to the Minister of Internal Affairs, Southern Rhodesia, 11th January, 1939.

[96] *Ibid.*

[97] *Ibid.*

The Medical Director concluded that the "cursory" medical examination of Africans was, at best, of extremely limited value. He argued that this method was only useful in detecting a small percentage of cases which without examination went undetected, but that "it has no value whatsoever as a crucial test enabling us [public health officials] to distinguish the infected from the non-infected and the infectious from the non-infectious."[98] The Medical Director suggested methods that were more effective than the one above and these included the adoption of (1) a tactile examination, that is, a thorough examination by the fingers of the examining officer, and (2) a series of highly technical laboratory tests such as the Wasserman Reaction (blood and cerebrospinal fluid tests) or microscopic examinations of smears and swabs. According to him, these methods often resulted in a reliable and accurate diagnosis in at least 90 percent of the cases.

However, these methods, though effective, were extremely difficult and costly to apply when dealing with large numbers of people. They also took a considerable amount of time. The collection of specimens for laboratory tests was slow and tedious so that the number of examinations that could be carried out by an examiner in an hour could be six at most. As a result, this method required employing many "medical men" to conduct the examinations at a high cost. In addition, the laboratory tests were complicated and time-consuming. With only two laboratories in Zimbabwe in 1939, one in Harare and the other one in Bulawayo, it was clear that this would require more spending and personnel.[99]

The lack of funds had also led to the mere treatment of symptoms of STDs without any attempt to cure them. Even treatment itself was costly. Each individual case cost approximately £1. Thus, the medical authorities could only focus on a method of treatment which relieved the patient of symptoms and rendering that patient non-infectious to others and this was achieved by administering a course of six injections given at the rate of one per week. Medical officials admitted that this treatment was largely a palliative one although it had the advantage of preventing the spread of infection.

What militated against the quick adoption of effective methods of medical examination was largely the lack of funding. However, the Medical Officer had more concerns about the application of these measures apart

[98] *Ibid.*
[99] *Ibid.*

from the question of finance. First, he was afraid that the introduction of a tactile examination would trigger great resentment particularly among African women.[100] He warned that these Africans were not coming to public health officials as sufferers seeking relief from pain and sickness, and for that reason, willing to undergo a certain amount of physical discomfort and embarrassment. On the contrary, these Africans were "being forced by the compulsion of law to submit themselves to an examination of an intimate character which for the most part they must consider totally unwarranted."[101] Second, the Medical Director doubted whether any government had the "moral right" to compel one section of the community to undergo a physical examination which was "repulsive to all its ideals" and one "***which was imposed merely for some dubious benefit which might or might not accrue to another section of the same community.***"[102] However, because the settler community was so powerful, the colonial government eventually implemented this detestable method. Thus, public health authorities instituted this system of tactile examination as a result of public pressure, although they themselves understood that these compulsory exams were ineffective in combating STDs. This clearly demonstrates what was wrong with public health in a colonial, undemocratic setting.

These European understandings of STDs in colonial Zimbabwe resembled those in South Africa and this was important because colonial Zimbabwe relied on South African laws as the basis for her own public health regulations. However, public health authorities in South Africa had already discredited these methods and were developing new ways of controlling STDs. In 1936 South African public health officials argued that although public interest in STDs continued, it was unfortunate that "this interest only too often expresses itself in demands and resolutions of an impracticable and ignorant nature."[103] The European community there had advocated wholesale compulsory examination and treatment, urging the government to introduce class and race discriminatory measures on non-European female servants and "prostitutes."[104] However, according

[100] *Ibid.*

[101] *Ibid.*

[102] *Ibid.* Emphasis added.

[103] *Ibid.*

[104] *Ibid.* For more on South African attempts to control the spread of STDs, see Jeremy C. Martens, "'Almost a Public Calamity': Prostitutes, 'Nurse Boys', and Attempts to Control Venereal Diseases in Colonial Natal, 1886–1890," *South African Historical Journal* 45 (2001): 27–52, E. van Heyningen, "The Social Evil in the Cape Colony, 1868–1902:

to the public health officials, such views revealed "the distorted attitude to venereal diseases of the large sections of the public." They suggested that wise education of the lay person as to the nature and extent of the problems of syphilis and gonorrhea could help in fostering an appreciation of the difficulties faced in controlling these diseases.

South African public health officials emphasized that compulsory examination and treatment of any section of the community, except in special circumstances, accomplished little. They warned that the definite diagnosis of even highly infectious phases might be extremely difficult and involve complicated laboratory technique. These South African officials also advised that a single examination could not be relied upon as a guarantee of freedom from infection for any length of time. Hence it was futile to attempt compulsory or heavy-handed methods of handling the problem.

Instead, officials in South Africa argued that the usual basis of successful programs of combating syphilis and gonorrhea was the provision of attractive and accessible treatment, administered with sympathetic consideration for the patient. In addition, they contended that because STDs in many stages were not superficially obvious, securing the trust and cooperation of the patient would stem out "the evil results of concealment." It was on this principle that the STD policy in South Africa was largely based by the 1930s. The South African Public Health Department therefore embarked upon securing free, convenient treatment in all areas through generous refunds on STD schemes instituted by local authorities.[105]

This South African report revealed a diversity of views within the European community. While the lay sections of the European community believed in the efficacy of compulsory medical examination of non-Europeans, the medical community in both South Africa and Zimbabwe argued that compulsory medical examinations were ineffective. This futility of public health policy toward STDs was another reason why Africans lacked trust in colonial public health.

However, despite all these concerns, colonial Zimbabwe eventually adopted the tactile system of medical examination, a system which some African women later referred to as *chibheura*, literally meaning being

Prostitution and the Contagious Diseases Acts," *Journal of Southern African Studies* 10, 2 (1984): 170–197, and R. Posel, "'Continental Women' and Durban's 'Social Evil,' 1899–1905," *Journal of Natal and Zulu History* 12 (1989).

[105] *Ibid.*

forced to open their legs for "inspection."[106] While there was some collusion in East Africa between British and Baganda male elite (particularly chiefs) on the need to control African women and their sexuality, this consensus is less evident in Southern Africa, perhaps because most of the chiefly powers had been usurped by colonial authorities under direct rule.[107] Even men resented these medical examinations. In Bulawayo, for instance, Africans disliked the "humiliation of medical examinations, when men were stripped naked."[108] One resident referred to the medical examination as a "disgrace" because this "show[ed] that the black man [was] an animal."[109]

With colonial officials placing the blame for the spread of STDs on unattached and mobile African women, compulsory STD examinations were a part of colonial regulations intended to control the mobility of Africans. While these medical examinations have been exclusively linked to influx controls in Zimbabwe, designed to limit the number of Africans entering European urban and mining spaces, there is danger of losing sight of the fact that these medical examinations were primarily public health initiatives aimed at preventing the spread of disease. Hence, medical examinations of Africans in general arose out of European fears of infection. Their premise was mistaken and racist, but this was the impetus for colonial public health policy.

Africans hated the invasive nature of these medical examinations. They also resented the medical examinations because they considered issues of sexual health to be private matters and in the past healers would have respected patients' preference not to expose bodies. Exposing bodies, particularly genitals would have been done only in the presence of the healer, unlike a hospital where STDs sufferers were exposed to nurses, attendants, and other patients. One elder, Mr. Mubekapi Matoro, said that to Africans

[106] For more on this, see Lynette A. Jackson, "'When in the White Man's Town': Zimbabwean Women Remember Chibeura," in *Women in African Colonial Histories*, ed. Jean Allman et al. (Indianapolis: Indiana University Press, 2002), 191–215.

[107] Vaughan, "Healing and Curing Issues," 132–136. Vaughan explains that the lack of control over women and their sexuality could threaten the male Baganda elites' control over marriage and kinship and by extension over the entire society. For the British, too, loss of control over female sexuality stood for and symbolized their inability to impose their control over African society in general.

[108] Terence Ranger, *Bulawayo Burning: The Social History of a Southern African City, 1893–1960* (James Currey: Suffolk, 2010), 49.

[109] *Ibid.*, 52.

STDs and menstrual problems were private matters. Going to the hospital with these diseases was a shameful act.[110]

In addition, some African men who had syphilis said that it showed manliness and perhaps a graduation into manhood. One interviewee from Penhalonga recalled, "Syphilis was common amongst the young men during our time [1940s and 50s] and you could boast of it but if you did not cure it, you could face serious consequences of paralysis or death if it got worse."[111] Asked if he was ever diagnosed of it, he responded,

> Oh yes it was my graduation into manhood. I was about twenty-something years old, just started working at Old West, and I had taken a woman from Nyaronga bar. I remember very well that it was her who caused it. I boasted to my friends but I could not be treated at the clinic I felt shy so I was treated by an old man we called him *Amankwala* (Chewa for medicine man).[112]

Africans therefore preferred to visit traditional doctors instead of violating their habits of discretion in relation to sexual relationships by going to hospitals and clinics. One interviewee noted,

> Venereal diseases were common but most young men did not report these because it meant a certain achievement to be sick of a minor and treatable venereal disease (they called it *siki*, referring to syphilis). I remember my friend who kept silent about this disease because his brother's wife worked at the mine clinic so she would get to hear of his problem if he sought treatment there. So he avoided the clinic until he could no longer walk properly and it was soon clear to everyone that he had a problem. Eventually, he was treated at the mine clinic.[113]

Thus, problems of STDs in African society went into the social realm of relations between youths and elders. While the elders did not necessarily disapprove of sexual activity by young people, they expected young people

[110] Interview with Mr. Mubekapi Matoro, Makubvu, Mozambique, 6 January, 2007.

[111] Interview, Penhalonga, Zimbabwe, 29 August, 2006.

[112] *Ibid*. This healer was probably a labor migrant from Malawi. On the causes of STDs, Edward Green has argued that Africans in central Mozambique understood syphilis to be caused by a common tiny, invisible, animate illness agent (*khoma*) or by direct contact with pus or other genital discharges (sometimes called dirt) that contain *khoma*. See Green, *Indigenous Theories of Contagious Disease*, 139.

[113] Interview, Tsvingwe Township, Penhalonga, Zimbabwe, 28 August, 2006.

to conduct their affairs with strict discretion so that these older people would not hear about them.

Another problem associated with medical examinations and treatment in hospitals and clinics was that government officials questioned the patients about how they contracted the disease. Officials forced patients to name every "contact," that is, a person they had sex with in order to track them down and treat them too. African STD patients therefore felt that colonial public health abused their habits of discretion in relation to sexual relationships. In contrast, African healers seldom questioned these patients about how they contracted STDs. As the same interviewee referenced above explained,

> [The doctors and nurses] at the clinic spoke the language that despised our understanding of health care. The nurses gave us a hard time. It was always our fault for getting sick even if it was a result of hard underground [mine] work. You see, that is why we went to *Amankwala* because he did not make a fuss about where we got syphilis, or to bring the person who gave it to us—such an embarrassing thing to do.[114]

Similar attitudes prevailed in other parts of Southern Africa. In South Africa, for example, an African male orderly, who served as a cultural broker between black hospital agents and a largely white medical staff at the Baragwaneth Hospital in Soweto, advised a junior white doctor in this way:

> You see, doctor, it's like this. When a patient goes to an African doctor [i.e., an indigenous healer] the doctor doesn't ask him a lot of funny questions about 'How do you feel? What is wrong with you? Where is the pain?' And so on. The doctor should know all about that. He can smell the sickness at once. What does take a long time is not the questions at the beginning but the treatment at the end—the mixtures and charms, the many things the patient is told to do or not to do. Very long instructions. But when the patient comes to the white doctor, the doctor asks him many, many questions about what he should know already. Then when it comes to the prescription the doctor only writes something very fast on a piece of paper, something you can't read even if you understand English. The [African] patient is not impressed with such things.[115]

[114] *Ibid*.

[115] Anne Digby, "Mid-Level Health Worker in South Africa: The In-Between Condition of the 'Middle,'" in *Public Health in the British Empire: Intermediaries, Subordinates, and the*

Hence, as mentioned earlier, colonial public health programs had limited success because colonial officials put little effort in understanding these cross-cultural matters.

Furthermore, while colonial officials blamed independent African women for the spread of STDs, Africans in Mozambique thought that soldiers, police, and government officials were the ones responsible for its spread. As Mr. Mubekapi Matoro recalled,

> This *Siki* [syphilis] was mainly spread by colonial soldiers who forced any woman, particularly girls to have unprotected sex with them. They left their victims with unwanted pregnancies and fatherless children. Locals tried to help girls by hiding them in caves, but it was of no use because the soldiers' movements were unpredictable.[116]

This concurs with the observations of the American Board missionaries at Mt. Selinda who reported that Portuguese colonial officials (*Commandants*) and their African policemen (*cipaes*) forcibly took concubines.[117] The missionaries claimed that although the *Commandant* at Spungabera was not involved in this practice, his two secretaries frequently developed sexual relationships with local African women in places where they worked. It was also the practice of these secretaries, "when out among the people collecting taxes, or in traveling thr[ough] the country, to demand native girls at night." Villagers therefore thought that all white men were the same. Thus, when the missionaries were out touring, they had to make it clear to villagers that they did not want to stay overnight and did not want girls. African communities had become so traumatized that all young unmarried girls fled upon hearing that some white men were coming.

In addition, the missionaries asserted that African "police boys," after the fashion of their white masters, also demanded girls whenever they liked and if a father denied the "police boy's" demand, the police boy soon found "something for which to accuse him before the Commandant as for instance to lie about his not having paid his tax or some other delinquency," which could result in a fine or being "sent away for work."[118]

Practice of Public Health, 1850–1960, ed. Ryan Johnson and Amna Khalid (Routledge: New York, 2012), 175.

[116] Interview with Mr. Mubekapi Matoro, Makubvu, Mozambique, 6 January, 2007.

[117] ABC 15.4, volume 33: Letter from J.R. Dysart, Gogoyo, P.E.A., to Dr. James L. Burton, Boston, MA, November 19, 1919.

[118] *Ibid*. Offenders could be sent to Beira to serve a long sentence with hard manual labor.

Conclusion

As this chapter has shown, cross-border movements had profound implications for the epidemiology of STDs, informing European attitudes toward Africans and influencing the formulation and implementation of public health policies in the region by exaggerating the risk of STDs introduced from Mozambique and other neighboring territories. Erroneous views on the epidemiology of STDs by the European settler community resulted in the adoption of discriminatory public health practices that singled out Africans for intrusive medical examinations.

Yet these public health measures, based on racial ideology, while constant and pervasive, were often ineffective. As shown in this chapter, medical examinations, performed in some cases by laymen without any medical background, were not effective. Yet regardless of whether or not these examinations were effective, they still interfered with the privacy and mobility of African men and women. Africans considered issues of sexual health a private matter. They preferred to deal with these issues in private, not by being forced to strip before total strangers or to name every person they had sexual intercourse with. Medical examinations therefore violated African norms of bodily modesty and discretion with regard to sexual relationships.

The permeability of the border also meant that public health policies in colonial Zimbabwe failed to stop the suspected diffusion of disease from Mozambique, widely regarded by colonial officials in Zimbabwe as a poorly governed reservoir of infection. In the end, erroneous understandings of the epidemiology of STDs by lay Europeans and the intrusiveness and ineffectiveness of compulsory medical examinations contributed to the lack of confidence in colonial public health among Africans.

References

Books, Articles, and Dissertations

Achola, Milcah Amolo. "The Public Health Ordinance Policy of the Nairobi Municipal/City Council 1945–62." In *African Historians and African Voices: Essays presented of Professor Bothwell Allan Ogot,* edited by E. S. Atieno Odhiambo. Basel: P. Schlettwein Publishing, 2001.

Digby, Anne. "Mid-Level Health Worker in South Africa: The In-between Condition of the 'Middle'." In *Public Health in the British Empire: Intermediaries, Subordinates, and the Practice of Public Health, 1850–1960*, edited by Ryan Johnson and Amna Khalid, 171–191. New York: Routledge, 2012.

Gelfand, Michael. *A Service to the Sick: A History of the Health Services for Africans in Southern Rhodesia, 1890–1953.* Gwelo: Mambo Press, 1976.

Green, Edward C. *Indigenous Theories of Contagious Disease.* Walnut Creek, CA: AltaMira Press, 1999.

Jeeves, Alan "Introduction: Histories of Reproductive Health and the Control of Sexually Transmitted Disease in Southern Africa: A Century of Controversy." *South African Historical Journal* 45 (2001): 1–10.

Lachenal, Guillaume. "A Genealogy of Treatment as Prevention (TasP): Prevention, Therapy, and the Tensions of Public Health in African History." In *Global Health in Africa: Historical Perspectives on Disease*, edited by L. A. James, J. R. Webb and Tamara Giles-Vernick, 70–91. Athens: Ohio University Press, 2013.

Levine, Philippa. *Prostitution, Race and Politics: Policing Venereal Disease in the British Empire.* New York: Routledge, 2003.

Martens, Jeremy C. "'Almost a Public Calamity': Prostitutes, 'Nurse Boys', and Attempts to Control Venereal Diseases in Colonial Natal, 1886–1890." *South African Historical Journal* 45 (2001): 27–52.

Packard, Randall M. *White Plague, Black Labor: Tuberculosis and the Political Economy of Health and Disease in South Africa.* Berkeley: University of California Press, 1989.

Posel, R. "'Continental Women' and Durban's 'Social Evil,' 1899–1905." *Journal of Natal and Zulu History* 12 (1989): 1–13.

Ranger, Terence. *Bulawayo Burning: The Social History of a Southern African City, 1893–1960.* Suffolk: James Currey, 2010.

Tuck, Michael W. "Kabaka Mutesa and Venereal Disease: An Essay on Medical History and Sources in Precolonial Buganda." *History in Africa* 30 (2003): 309–325.

Vambe, Lawrence. *From Rhodesia to Zimbabwe.* Pittsburgh: University of Pittsburgh Press, 1976.

van Heyningen, E. "The Social Evil in the Cape Colony, 1868–1902: Prostitution and the Contagious Diseases Acts." *Journal of Southern African Studies* 10, 2 (1984): 170–197.

van Onselen, Charles. *Chibaro: African Mine Labour in Southern Rhodesia, 1900–1933.* London: Pluto Press, 1976.

Vasse, Guillaume. "The Mozambique Company's Territory II." *Journal of the Royal African Society* 6, 24 (1907): 385–389.

Vaughan, Megan. "Syphilis in Colonial East and Central Africa: The Social Construction of an Epidemic." In *Epidemics and Ideas: Essays on the Historical Perception of Pestilence*, edited by Terence Ranger and Paul Slack, 269–302. Cambridge: Cambridge University Press, 1992.

Vaughan, Megan. *Curing Their Ills: Colonial Power and African Illness.* Stanford: Stanford University Press, 1993.

Vaughan, Megan. "Healing and Curing Issues in the Social History and Anthropology of Medicine in Africa." *Social History of Medicine* 7, 2 (1994): 283–295.

Webster, M. H. "A Review of the Development of the Health Services of Rhodesia from 1923 to the Present Day, Part I, the 1920s." *The Central African Journal of Medicine* 18, 12 (December, 1972): 244–247.

CHAPTER 8

Borders and the Provision of Health Services for Rural Africans

This chapter is about various kinds of borders. It considers the colonial border, the rural and urban border, the border between whites and blacks, the border between public health and curative medicine, as well as the border between Western biomedicine and African medicine and how these borders influenced the provision of health care. An exploration of the border between public health and curative medicine and their reception by Africans at the site of the clinic and hospital shows that African societies were dynamic and willing to experiment with certain aspects of colonial medicine. This examination also reveals the different tiers of health care provision that represented and reproduced colonial ideologies of racism, coercion, paternalism, and control. In the urban and mining centers there were more hospitals and clinics than in the rural areas. There was thus a disparity in health provision between rural and urban settings. However, racial discrimination was the norm across the board, with the best facilities being reserved for European settlers. There was also a disparity in health care provision between Mozambique and Zimbabwe, meaning that Africans in Mozambique and even whites crossed the border to seek health services in Zimbabwe, raising the perennial fears of diffusion of disease. Moreover, this chapter also makes the distinction between missionary and state medicine, arguing that missionary medicine, with its out-patient and self-administered orientation, was received much more enthusiastically and embraced by Africans than the restrictive and controlled setting of colonial hospitals. Thus, contrary to popular belief, Africans were not distrustful of

F. Dube, *Public Health at the Border of Zimbabwe and Mozambique, 1890–1940*, African Histories and Modernities,
https://doi.org/10.1007/978-3-030-47535-2_8

Western medicine *per se*; they were distrustful of the methods of its delivery and what those methods represented and reproduced, that is, racism, coercion, paternalism, and control.

As far as the development of health services for Africans in the colonies is concerned, the standard narrative has been that curative services were largely left to missionaries, with the exception of the medical care that was provided to urban employees in the early years of colonial rule.[1] However, in the post-First World War period, continues the narrative, while still mostly concerned with the reproduction of a healthy labor force, colonial officials gave African health more attention, but this was still a half-hearted approach which continued in the late 1920s and in the 1930s. This was a culmination of calls from some colonial circles and African peoples for improvement in socio-economic conditions and for a focus on "African welfare." Still, the dearth of political will ensured that only a handful of these initiatives were sustained.[2] These developments of the 1920s and 1930s were then followed by the development of vaccinations and antibodies as well as the increasing calls by indigenous peoples for better living standards and for political participation, which led to the extension of health care to the larger society in the 1940s, particularly in the British and French colonies.[3] Hence, after the Second World War, Britain introduced "development" and "welfare" acts in its colonies, partly inspired by self-interest but also by more "progressive," albeit paternalistic, notions of colonial trusteeship, in which government planning and investment would promote economic and social progress.[4] The same could not be said, however, about Belgian and Portuguese colonies in Africa, as well as South

[1] Prince, "Introduction: Situating Health and the Public in Africa," 17. See also Michael, Worboys, "The Colonial World as Mission and Mandate: Leprosy and Empire, 1900–1940," *Osiris* 15, 1 (2000): 207–219.

[2] Ibid., 18. See also Randall Packard, "Visions of Postwar Health and Development and Their Impact on Public Health Interventions in the Developing World," in *Internal Development and the Social Sciences: Essays on the History and Politics of Knowledge*, ed. Fredrick Cooper and Randall Packard (Berkeley: University of California Press, 1997), 93–115.

[3] Ibid. See also Packard, "Visions of Postwar Health and Development," and Joanna Lewis, *Empire State-Building: War And Welfare In Kenya 1925–52* (Athens: Ohio University Press, 2001), and Helen Tilley, *Africa as a Living Laboratory: Empire, Development, and the Problem of Scientific Knowledge, 1870–1950* (Chicago: University of Chicago Press, 2011).

[4] Ibid. See also Lewis, *Empire State-Building*, 79, 86, 105.

Africa and Zimbabwe, which did not care much about the welfare of Africans.[5]

A recent study in pre-apartheid South Africa has revealed that medical practitioners did not always follow the biomedical ideal of ethical and impartial treatment of patients because they sometimes acted in the interests of commercial and political players.[6] This connivance of medical authority and colonial capital resulted in perilous health decisions, for example, doctors being used to play down the threat of a smallpox outbreak in order to maintain the flow of African labor to the Kimberley diamond mines, critical for the growth of white capital.[7] Similar collusion between medicine and capital is also evident in introduction of contraceptives to colonial farms in Zimbabwe in the 1960s, which was driven more by white farmers' interest in maximizing their workforce's efficiency and output than by concerns for African laborers' health and well-being.[8] Yet even where attempts to improve living conditions of Africans and promote development were made, these efforts remained apathetic, sporadic, and incomplete and mostly focused on appeasing the most politically vociferous groups, such as urban wage laborers in the hope of demoralizing political protest.[9]

This chapter deviates from this traditional narrative and instead focuses on the second category of colonies, where very little was done to improve the health conditions of Africans, including Portuguese East Africa and Zimbabwe. Although some colonial officials argued that the creation of hospitals and clinics for Africans was driven by genuine concern for the health of Africans, the history of rural health services in Mozambique and Zimbabwe suggests that this was the last line of defense for the colonial

[5] Ibid., 45.

[6] Russell Stafford Viljoen, "Disease, Doctors and De beers Capitalists: Smallpox and Scandal in Colonial Kimberley (South Africa) during the Mineral Revolutions and British Imperialism, c. 1882–1883," in *Biomedicine as a Contested Site: Some Revelations in Imperial Contexts*, ed. Poonam Bala (Lanham, MD: Lexington Books, 2009), 158.

[7] Ibid.

[8] Amy Kaler, "The White Man in the Bedroom: Contraception and Resistance on Commercial Farms in Colonial Rhodesia," in *Biomedicine as a Contested Site: Some Revelations in Imperial Contexts*, ed. Poonam Bala (Lanham, MD: Lexington Books, 2009), 80.

[9] Ibid., 18. See also Frederick Cooper, *Africa since 1940: The Past of the Present*, (Cambridge: Cambridge University Press, 2002), 43–44, 85, and Andrew Burton and Michael Jennings, "The Emperor's New Clothes?: Continuities in Governance in Late Colonial and Early Post colonial East Africa," *International Journal of African Historical Studies* 40, 1 (2007): 1–25.

society against disease. This partially explains why these services came relatively late in the colonial period, in the 1930s, after the realization that the best form of safeguarding the health of the white settler community was to treat diseases in Africans. In Zimbabwe, in particular, the decision to create a rural health infrastructure was a culmination of economic imperatives and settlers' fears of "infectious natives" spreading diseases to the white settler community. Provision of health services for rural Africans, therefore, served as a public health strategy of treatment as prevention.[10] In the border region of Mozambique, by contrast, the lack of a rural health service reflected a weaker settler influence on government.

However, even in areas they were established, these government health services for rural Africans reflected the conventional thinking of Western medical professionals at the time that hospital confinement was the best form of treatment.[11] This approach caused problems of two kinds. First, insistence on hospitalization contradicted African views on the best ways of treating many afflictions. As a result, just as public health measures caused hardship, harassment, prosecution, and imprisonment, the delivery of government curative health services caused resentment because it failed to accommodate African treatment preferences and concepts of illness. Second, the expense of this approach meant that the coverage of rural African communities by government health services remained limited. In the absence of government curative services, therefore, in many rural areas Western biomedicine was left to missionaries. In the southern part of the Zimbabwe-Mozambique border region, it was the American Board of Commissioners for Foreign Missions (American Board Mission) at Mt. Selinda and Chikore, as well as Gogoyo in Mozambique, which provided rural curative medical services. These missionaries, while still condemning "traditional" medicine, were more flexible in accommodating African preference for out-patient treatment because their primary goal was to win converts. They were less insistent on hospitalization and more willing to make visits to patients' homes and distribute medicine. However, the border restricted their work and consequently became an obstacle to their work.

[10] For a detailed discussion of treatment as prevention, see Lachenal, "A Genealogy of Treatment as Prevention (TasP)."

[11] Even in the West, confinement and observation was emphasized in treating infections. Michel Foucault has emphasized these aspects, see Michel Foucault, *Discipline and Punish: The Birth of the Prison* (New York: Vintage Books, 1995).

An examination of rural health care in the Zimbabwe-Mozambique border shows that although Africans often rejected public health measures, they responded quite differently to the provision of treatment services. African societies were innovative, open to new ways of healing, and willing to test alternatives. Curiosity and dissatisfaction with established healing methods led to willingness to try alternatives. Yet, although Africans were willing to try out curative services, they disliked confinement in hospitals, where they lost control over the healing process. Their dislike of hospitalization stemmed from one of the principal precolonial views of healing which granted patients and their families a high degree of control over healing. Precolonial healing was often best done in a patient's home or community, where patient had access to multiple therapeutic alternatives and advice from kin and where practitioners could get detailed knowledge of the social relationships which might affect a patient's health. In some cases, however, this precolonial healing was not strictly confined to a patient's immediate surroundings, because sometimes, particularly in cases involving spirits or physical ailments, patients left their homes to visit specialists. The same trend developed among African Independent Churches (AICs) after their introduction to Zimbabwe in the 1920s.

In stark contrast to the versatile repertoire of methods and close attention to social conditions practiced in precolonial healing, colonial government health services were rigid and neglected social circumstances. Due to the fact that most rural Africans had not received a Western education, colonial officials believed that the only effective way of treating them was through confinement and close supervision by European physicians in hospitals. Hence, the mode of delivery of government treatment services did not respond to African preferences. Even the establishment of rural dispensaries (out-patient treatment centers) by colonial governments in the late 1930s was a result of financial considerations, not African preferences.

African understandings of illness and healing help to explain why Africans favored missionary medicine. Missionaries not only visited the sick in their homes but also more eagerly provided out-patient services to those who visited their hospitals and clinics than government hospitals. These practices meant that Africans often used Western medicines with limited European supervision. As a result, medical missionaries and government officials complained that Africans misused Western medicines, particularly by combining them with indigenous pharmacopeia. Yet this, too, reflected the enduring strength of the tradition of experimentation with alternative therapies, as did African insistence on sharing their understandings of disease and healing with missionaries.

In the southern part of the Zimbabwe-Mozambique border region, the center of missionary medical services was a station established by the American Board Mission at Mt. Selinda in 1893. Owing to the fact that, at that time, supervision of the border barely existed, the American Board missionaries assumed that they could extend health care throughout a catchment area that included territory in both Zimbabwe and Mozambique. When the border was officially demarcated in 1899, however, they faced new difficulties. Much of their catchment area had fallen into the Mozambican side while the mission station was on the Zimbabwean side. Yet it was vital for them to cover the entire area because, given that their primary goal was evangelization, they had a strong incentive to accommodate African preferences by extending their medical practice into local communities. They felt that providing medical services in ways which accommodated African understandings of illness and healing would be the best way to lure Africans to Christianity. Their need to accommodate African preferences led them to ignore government restrictions on border crossings and government insistence on confining African patients in hospitals. In this way, missionary encounters were two-way processes, where both the missionaries and Africans shaped historical processes.[12]

By contrast, as colonial governments became concerned with the "public health threats" posed by "infective natives," they dismissed African healing preferences while asserting their own theories of disease and healing. Even Portuguese officials who had formerly tolerated hybridization of healing practices now shifted to outright rejection and repression of indigenous healing practices at the end of the nineteenth century.[13] Hence, among the Portuguese in Mozambique, there emerged a clear distinction between what Europeans considered proper (European) and improper (indigenous) medical practices, as the Portuguese dismissed indigenous healing practices as "savage, primitive, superstitious and ignorant, rude, vile, and dirty."[14]

[12] For a more in-depth discussion of missionary encounters, see Dube, "Medicine without Borders."

[13] Bastos, "Medical Hybridisms and Social Boundaries," 768.

[14] Ibid.

Inspired by these views, colonial governments in both Mozambique and Zimbabwe interfered with precolonial healing and public health practices such as rain-making and identification of sorcerers. For example, the 1899 Witchcraft Suppression Act in Zimbabwe did much, thought American Board missionaries, to break down a "powerful impediment in the upward progress of the nation."[15] When famine struck as a result of drought in Gogoyo, Mozambique, in 1916, another American Board missionary reported that a rain doctor complained that he could not practice because of government interference.[16]

During the early years of colonial rule, therefore, rural Africans found themselves between a rock and a hard place. They found that they had only limited access to hospitals and clinics at a time when colonial rule had weakened their own public health and healing systems. However, in the 1920s the growing political influence of settlers and increasing pleas by Western-educated Africans led to the extension of health services to Africans in rural areas. The colonial government in Zimbabwe established a network of dispensaries in the rural areas to provide treatment services to Africans. In Mozambique, however, where settler influence was weaker, the Portuguese established a much less extensive rural health infrastructure, which relied heavily on the provision of medical services through schools.

Nevertheless, the dominant narrative by colonial officials in both territories was that colonialism greatly improved a lot of colonized Africans. These officials argued that Western biomedicine reduced sickness in African populations, causing a sharp decline in mortality. Thus colonial officials often touted "Proud Record" or "Tropical Victory," particularly in their assessment of the impact of Western medicine on Zimbabwe, Zambia, and Malawi.[17] Yet, prior to 1918, colonial governments did not do much to establish rural health services.[18] While financial constraints played a huge role in the lop-sided development of health services, the primary factor was colonial priorities. Emphasis on European health and

[15] Smith, *A History of the American Board Missions in Africa*, 41. The Witchcraft Suppression Act made it a crime to accuse someone of being a witch.

[16] American Board of Commissioners for Foreign Missions Archives, Boston, MA, U.S.A. (hereafter, ABC) 15.4, volume 32: Letter from Dr. W. T. Lawrence, Mt. Silinda, Melsetter, Rhodesia, South Africa, May 13th, 1916.

[17] Michael Gelfand, *Proud Record in Health Services in Rhodesia and Nyasaland* (Salisbury, Southern Rhodesia, 1959).

[18] Packard, "Visions of Postwar Health and Development," 94.

economic well-being dictated where resources were spent, and it was not on African health. What most rural inhabitants encountered were the coercive public health programs, such as smallpox campaigns, not the curative services that they—particularly those who had been "enlightened" by Western education—were willing to try. Therefore, African societies were open to innovation, but the nature of colonial health services discouraged the adoption of biomedicine. Hence the eradication of African "superstition" and the application of "science" and "reason" to the colonized were colonial goals which were never fully realized.

Health Services for Rural Africans, 1890–1930

African health services in both Mozambique and Zimbabwe suffered neglect from colonial governments up to the 1930s. While officials at the top of the colonial government preferred hospitals, those on the ground complained about complete lack of health services. This preference for hospitals impeded the creation of a less-expensive system of treatment delivery. In Mozambique, in August 1904 the administrator of the Mossurize district remarked upon the need for medical services at Spungabera in the southern part of the border region, a concern he had raised earlier in 1902.[19] As a clear indication of preference for treatment of Africans in hospitals, the Director of Medical Services for the Mozambique Company urged the government to construct new wards in existing African hospitals.[20]

In Zimbabwe, as late as 1924, the colonial government did not have a scheme for the treatment of Africans, a testimony to the fact that medical services were originally for European settlers only. There were some facilities in urban areas and only a few medical units under the control of mission stations operating in rural areas. These facilities "were, however, totally inadequate and in actual fact, very little was being done to meet the essential medical needs of Natives."[21] In 1924, Reverend G. Hardaker of

[19] AHM, FCM, Secretaria Geral—Relatórios: Relatório mensal da circunscrição de Mossurize, Agosto, 1904, Caixa 259.

[20] AHM, FCM, Secretaria Geral—Relatórios: Relatório da Direcção dos Serviços de Saúde, 1928, Caixa 116, Pasta 2283.

[21] NAZ, S2803/FNWS/63: Internal Affairs-Health, 1941 August 5–1948 February 3, Memorandum-Federation of Native Welfare Societies in Southern Rhodesia: National Health Services for Africans, 6th September, 1942.

the Southern Rhodesia Missionary Conference pleaded with the Medical Director for medical assistance to Africans:

> In our journeys on the Reserves all Missionaries see cases of unnecessary suffering. We do what we can, in our simple way, to help, but we feel that the Government might also do something more than it is doing at present. Dispensaries within reach of every Reserve (whether under Gov[ernment] or Missionary control) would be a means of great help. At a recent meeting of native teachers[,] a pathetic plea was brought forward for help, and the remark was made by a native that the Gov[ernment] provided medicine for all their (the natives') cattle (alluding to Dips) but not for the people.[22]

It is important to note that this "pathetic plea" from African teachers was a request to the government to distribute medicines on an out-patient basis, just as the missionaries did. This plea also came from African teachers who had received a Western education and therefore more likely to appreciate Western ways. That the colonial government provided treatment for African-owned cattle in the form of dip tanks while not doing enough to alleviate the suffering of the people was not surprising at all. One of the goals of colonialism was to exploit the colonies for the benefit of the mother countries. The cattle industry was, together with tobacco and maize farming, the most productive sectors of the Zimbabwean economy. The only Africans who got modest medical care were those employed on farms, plantations or by mining companies because the employers wished to maintain a stable and healthy workforce and also wished to prevent the spread of diseases to Europeans from Africans who they regarded as the "reservoir of infection." In addition to the importance of cattle to the economy, ideas of bovine diseases paralleled those of human diseases in that Europeans made dipping of African-owned cattle mandatory not so much because they wanted to preserve African wealth, but because they feared the spread of disease to their own herds.

The breakthrough in the extension of health services to Africans in Zimbabwe's rural areas came when chartered BSAC rule ended in 1923 and Colonial Zimbabwean settlers chose "Responsible Government." This arrangement gave settlers considerable autonomy from Britain. Settlers now had the means to implement legislative changes to their own

[22] NAZ, S1173/301–304: Medical Missions, 1924–1932, Rev. G. Hardaker, Southern Rhodesia Missionary Conference, to the Medical Director, Southern Rhodesia, 21st June 1924.

benefit. The European settler community dreaded the spread of diseases from Africans, whom it considered to be reservoirs of infection. The settler community argued that the best way to safeguard their own health and have a healthy African labor force was through treating infectious diseases in Africans.

However, the Public Health Department in Zimbabwe still confronted four difficulties, which, according to Percy Ibbotson of the Federation of Native Welfare Societies in Zimbabwe, were the inadequacy of existing medical facilities, the lack of training for African orderlies, the scattered nature of the African population distribution, and African opposition to "European medicine."[23] However, although Africans generally resented preventative public health programs, they were willing to try curative forms which gave them some form of control over treatment. In the Zimbabwe-Mozambique border region the NC Mutare reported in 1924 that Africans appeared to have overcome their apathy to hospital treatment and that several of them had sought treatment, "so much so that some had to be turned away for lack of accommodation."[24] In the same year, the NC Chipinge also reported, "Natives sometimes *request* to be sent to the Government Medical Officer for treatment."[25]

In 1926 the NC Chipinge went further to state that the women who resided within the reach of the doctor at Mt. Selinda or the nurse in charge at Chikore Mission Station could no longer be "contented with the superstitious mouthings of the old crones who attend as midwives but clamour for the help which they have learnt to appreciate and for which they appear to be really grateful."[26] Although his comment reflected a disdainful attitude of colonial officials toward African practices, it also demonstrates African willingness to experiment with Western medicine.

However, government health services for Africans in rural areas were still non-existent. In the 1920s there was only one government hospital in

[23] NAZ, S2803/FNWS/63: Internal Affairs-Health, 1941 August 5–1948 February 3, Memorandum-Federation of Native Welfare Societies in Southern Rhodesia: National Health Services for Africans, 6th September, 1942.

[24] NAZ, S235/502: Report of the Native Commissioner, Umtali District, for the Year ended 31st December, 1924.

[25] NAZ, S235/502: Report of the Native Commissioner, Melsetter District, for the Year ended 31st December, 1924. Italics reflect my emphasis.

[26] NAZ, S235/502: Report of the Native Commissioner, Melsetter District, for the Year ended 31st December, 1926. This was a reference to the medical services of the American Board Mission which established hospitals at Mt. Selinda and Chikore.

Mutare, an urban center, and several missionary hospitals at Mutambara, Rusitu, Chikore, and Mt. Selinda. In 1929 several chiefs petitioned for the establishment of dispensaries in their reserves.[27] A report of the NC Mutare commented on the circumstances which led to this petition:

> During my patrols I noted several diseases such as Ophthalmia which should be treated locally. Not only does the education of the children suffer but the labour supply of the country is seriously diminished through insufficient medical attention.[28]

The prominence of the labor question in health initiatives for Africans is clearly evident in the statement above. However, while members of the settler community and missionaries pressed for reform, government physicians took the lead in justifying the extension of health services to Africans. Their primary concern was the health of European settlers. One of these physicians, Dr. Askins, then the Medical Director of Zimbabwe, argued, "Here we have an extraordinarily healthy country for white people to live in, but on the whole our death rate is not as low as it ought to be considering the young constitution of the population, *and as we want to have a healthy white population we have got to tackle infectious diseases in the native.*"[29] He went on to argue that Africans were the reservoir of these infectious diseases and that, "Take malaria. No amount of nets and screens will prevent it in a country like this unless measures are taken to deal with it in the native. Take dysentery. Most of our dysentery comes from native carriers."[30] Thus treating infections among Africans was not an end in itself but a means to an end, the end being the health of European settlers! Referring to a speech by a government minister who had used the economic aphorism that "the best way to increase your own wealth is to increase the wealth of those around you," Askins argued in similar terms that the "best way to increase your own health is to increase the health of those around you."[31]

[27] NAZ, S235/507: Report of the Native Commissioner, Umtali District for the year ended the 31st December, 1929.

[28] Ibid., Ophthalmia is inflammation of the eye.

[29] NAZ, S1173/336: Scheme for Medical Treatment of Natives, by Dr. Askins, Medical Director, Southern Rhodesia, 1930. Emphasis added.

[30] Ibid.

[31] Ibid.

The fear of spread of diseases from the African population to the Europeans was enough to guarantee swift action. In 1930 medical officials further emphasized the urgency of such a move, noting that beyond a small amount of hospital treatment and a few cases brought forward by the NCs, the government was doing little for the medical needs of 950,000 Africans in colonial Zimbabwe.[32] Askins clearly articulated this fear when he reported that most of the diseases that occurred in endemic or epidemic form among Africans were liable to spread to Europeans. Askins tried to heighten the impression of danger by highlighting the high rates of infant mortality which prevailed among Africans. He cited a "highly experienced NC in the Southern Rhodesia Service" who told him that more than half of African babies born in colonial Zimbabwe died within one year.[33] Askins used such claims of the prevalence of childhood diseases to argue that as long as these diseases existed, they could spread to the European community.

Advancing his case for medical treatment of Africans, Askins reiterated the concerns of many settlers that diseases supposedly prevalent among Africans could spread into the European community. He argued that throughout the African population of Zimbabwe, there were "to be found many extreme examples of Africans in the late stages of such diseases as leprosy, yaws, etc." He argued that infection could be conveyed to European households by African carriers, who, to all outward appearances. looked perfectly well.[34] Other infections which Askins cited as potential dangers were malaria, dysentery, internal worms (hookworm), bilharzia (schistosomiasis), venereal disease, cerebrospinal meningitis, smallpox, and sleeping sickness.

The high incidence of some of these infections in the European population encouraged the belief that they originated from the African population. Malaria, for example, was the chief preventable cause of death among European babies and children of school age in Zimbabwe.[35] Medical

[32] Ibid.

[33] NAZ, S1173/336: Preliminary Report on the Medical Treatment of Natives, R.A. Askins, Medical Director, Southern Rhodesia, 8th September, 1930. The fact that the Medical Director relied on anecdotal evidence from an NC demonstrated government failure to collect reliable statistics. Indeed, the government only recorded vital statistics for Europeans in its public health reports. The only data on the African population came from crude estimates of NCs.

[34] Ibid.

[35] Ibid.

officials also asserted that Africans spread strains of amoebic and bacillary dysentery to Europeans, causing "much suffering." These officials asserted that cerebrospinal meningitis was common among Africans and was usually borne to European households by apparently healthy African carriers.[36]

Erroneous views about the epidemiology of diseases heightened fears of infections. For example, in the case of venereal diseases, the common assumption was that all Africans were infected with syphilis as demonstrated earlier. Even professionals such as physicians sometimes succumbed to lay settler fears and distortion of established facts. For instance, medical officials in colonial Zimbabwe were concerned that although venereal syphilis was infectious almost entirely through the medium of sexual intercourse it was "undesirable from an aesthetic point of view that there should be the risk of native boys being employed in European houses whilst they are suffering from this disease." They asserted that infection through other means than sexual intercourse, "though exceedingly rare," was "nevertheless possible."[37]

Europeans also held erroneous ideas about human trypanosomiasis, which supposedly threatened the health of Europeans. "[Currently], many authorities doubt the importance of big game as a factor in the maintenance of human trypanosomiasis in tsetse areas," Askins wrote. "[I]t is possible that infected natives are the cause of the disease remaining endemic in certain of such districts."[38] He claimed that in any district where the *Glossina morsitans* (tsetse) fly was common there was "always a grave possibility of an epidemic of sleeping sickness in the event of an outbreak being started by infective natives." In actual fact, wild animals were the major reservoirs of this disease. Provision of medical services to Africans was therefore partly driven by erroneous understandings of epidemiology.

At the insistence of physicians, missionaries, NCs, and the settler community, the colonial government began to look deeper into African health issues. Its approach was shaped by a tendency to dismiss African understandings of illness and healing and to insist upon European supervision of medical treatment. In 1924, A. M. Fleming, then Medical Director, expressed his preference for the treatment of Africans in hospitals under European supervision by saying that as far as the needs for sick Africans

[36] Ibid.
[37] Ibid.
[38] Ibid.

were concerned, ample provision was made in hospitals.[39] In response to the requests to provide medical aid to Africans in rural areas, the government took a two-pronged approach. One of the approaches involved a scheme of dispensaries or "collection centers" managed by the colonial government. The seriously sick would be "collected" at these centers for transfer to hospitals. The other approach involved placing the responsibility for African medical care on the missionaries. This was in effect a continuation of the previous strategy, the only difference being that the colonial government now gave grants to missionary societies providing medical attention to Africans in reserves. These approaches resembled schemes undertaken in other British territories such as Kenya, Uganda, and Tanzania after 1920.[40]

First Approach: Dispensaries in African Reserves

Under this approach, the colonial government in Zimbabwe built dispensaries in African reserves under the aegis of the African Affairs Department. The major feature of this scheme involved plotting out the colony into districts, with each district having its own central hospital surrounded by a ring of dispensaries not exceeding six in number and not more distant than 50 miles on motorable roads.[41] Each dispensary would treat Africans from a radius of approximately 75 miles or a diameter of 150 miles.

Staffed by an African orderly as a caretaker and dresser, these centers "gathered" the sick at designated points in the African reserves where they could be visited periodically by the local government medical officer.[42] Medical officials indicated that the seriously ill could be transferred to the nearest Government Hospital for special care and treatment.

[39] NAZ, S1173/328–329: A. M. Fleming, Medical Director, Southern Rhodesia, to the Colonial Secretary, 25th June, 1924.

[40] David Baronov, *The African Transformation of Western Medicine and the Dynamics of Global Cultural Exchange* (Philadelphia: Temple University Press, 2008), 115–119.

[41] NAZ, S1173/336: "Scheme for the Medical Treatment of Natives", R.A. Askins, Medical Director, to the Chief Native Commissioner, Southern Rhodesia, 24th December, 1930.

[42] NAZ, S1173/328–329: Medical Assistance to Indigenous Natives in Reserves, Medical Director, Southern Rhodesia, to The Secretary, Department of the Colonial Secretary, Southern Rhodesia, 9th June, 1927.

Colonial officials continued to refine the scheme for the medical treatment of Africans over the years. In October 1930 they proposed to establish a number of stations where there would be a government medical officer, an African hospital, an out-patient department, and a small nursing staff, in addition to creating a ring of African dispensaries around each station.[43] In order to staff these centers, the colonial government planned to train male African orderlies and possibly female African nurses in larger African hospitals. A proposed government maternity training school would be responsible for training African midwives.

After launching this program in the 1930s, by 1946, Zimbabwe had 76 clinics or rural hospitals. Colonial officials reported that "Africans had become accustomed to them and were coming there unhesitatingly and entrusting their children to the clinic staff" and that maternity facilities had been added and were "very popular."[44] The sick were examined and admitted to the clinics from where those acutely ill were transferred by ambulance to nearest main urban center at Harare, Bulawayo, Gweru, Mutare, Masvingo, Kwekwe, Kadoma, Rusape, or Bindura where "modern" medical, surgical, and obstetrical facilities had been established. Unlike mission hospitals which made a "small charge" for treatment, all services including hospitalization were free in government hospitals and the claim was made again that "so popular" had the clinics become that in 1948 Dr. Morris, then the Medical Director, was afraid that the Health Department would be inundated with requests for new ones. As a result, the Health Department decided that no clinics would be built within a 20-mile radius from existing medical facilities. Again, officials claimed that Africans were now using the rural hospitals for "normal confinements" and that at all the clinics female nursing orderlies were stationed to perform maternity work and, even at some, male orderlies were enjoying much local esteem for this service.[45] This reflected the willingness among Africans to experiment with Western medicine. Similar trends were evident in other colonies around this time. In East Africa Western education and colonial jobs from the early 1930s contributed to a change in the critique of Western biomedicine, from whether to accept or reject biomedicine to what to embrace and how to institutionalize what was

[43] NAZ, S1173/336: Treatment of Natives, R.A. Askins, Medical Director, to the Secretary, Department of the Colonial Secretary, Southern Rhodesia, 31st October, 1930.

[44] Gelfand, *A Service to the Sick*, 128.

[45] Ibid., 129.

embraced.[46] In much of colonial Africa, this shift, however, was not driven by the need for "social betterment," because this social betterment lay not in Western biomedicine supplanting Africans healing practices, as envisioned by the colonial state, but rather in embracing certain aspects of Western biomedicine while retaining certain core African therapeutics.[47]

While reports such as the ones quoted above present a picture of extensive health facilities for Africans, the reality was that as late as 1952, there was little improvement in health services over the situation that had existed in the 1930s. In Chimanimani district, for instance, the NC reported in 1952 that there were only "two modern" clinics in the sub-district.[48] This was in addition to the Rusitu and Mutambara mission clinics. As a result of this lack of medical facilities, some Africans traveled distances of more than 25 miles in order to get to the nearest treatment center. These few treatment centers served an African population of 23,960 in 1952.

Another indication that government health services for Africans were inadequate was evident in the report of the NC Chimanimani, who reported that only those living near clinics took the trouble to seek health care because transport facilities virtually did not exist.[49] In the south the NC of Chipinge district, with about 51,213 Africans, reported that the Chipinge Native Clinic was inadequate to meet the growing demands for health care. He said:

> The Chipinga Native Clinic has worked at full pressure during the year. Although urgent minor repairs have been done the clinic is still in a bad state of repair. A Native Hospital should be built, as Chipinga serves as a base for all the outside clinics and all serious surgical and medical cases are sent in. Accommodation is limited. If a fully equipped native hospital could be erected the European nursing and secretarial staff could assist in the administration.[50]

[46] Ndege, *Health, State, and Society in Kenya*, p. 10.

[47] Ibid., See Ann Beck, *A Medical History of the British Medical Administration of East Africa, 1900–1950* (Cambridge: Harvard University Press, 1970).

[48] NAZ, S2827/2/2/2 Annual Report of the Assistant Native Commissioner, Melsetter, for the Year ended 31st December, 1952.

[49] Ibid.

[50] NAZ, S2403/2681: Native Commissioners' Reports, 1952, Report of the Native Commissioner, Chipinga, for the year ended 31st December, 1952.

Clearly, these medical services for Africans were not enough. To the west of Chipinge, the Save Valley was served by two clinics only, Birchenough and Nyanyadzi.[51] The NC added that the majority of the African population lived south of this area, which was not served by a clinic.

In the northern part of the Zimbabwe-Mozambique border region, the clinics at St. Augustine's Mission, Old Mutare Mission, in the Marange Reserve, Odzi Village, and Tsonzo Division were inadequate for an African population of 86,506 in 1959 in rural Mutare district as these clinics were "invariably overcrowded."[52] Reflecting the African preference for out-patient treatment, these hospitals and clinics gave "innumerable outpatient treatments." The NC Mutare noted that "additional curative institutions" would be warranted in his district, especially in the Muromo Special Native Area and the Mutasa North Reserve, where the medical facilities provided by the Ziwe Zano Society at the Honde Clinic continued to be inadequate and unsatisfactory.[53]

Reflecting the enduring reliance of government on the medical services of religious institutions, in 1961 the Roman Catholic Mission opened a clinic at Chisumbanje, south of Chipinge. This clinic was staffed "by European nurses, one an American and one a Canadian."[54] It improved what, according to the NC Chipinge, was a desperate position for the African population, but was still small and inadequate. Apart from this clinic, the only other option for sick African residents of southern Chipinge district was a small, informal clinic run out of her house by the wife of the Land Development Officer at Chibuwe. In addition, the American Board Mission ran an out-patient center at Zamuchiya, some 28 miles south of Chikore Mission Station. Reliance on these mission health centers clearly demonstrated the inadequacy of government services, which is the subject of the following section.

[51] Ibid.

[52] NAZ, S2827/2/2/7: Annual Report of the Native Commissioner, Umtali, for the Year ended 31st December, 1959.

[53] Ibid. The Ziwe Zano Society was an indigenous African society.

[54] NAZ, S2827/2/2/8: Annual Report of the Native Commissioner, Chipinga, for the Year ended 31st December, 1961. Note that Americans and Canadians were considered "European" in this case.

Second Approach: Provision of Medical Assistance Through Missionary Societies

Apart from government health services, colonial governments sought to extend health services to Africans through religious institutions. Mission medical work for Africans in Zimbabwe was started by Dr. Edward Rundle of the Anglican Mission in Mutare, who settled in Chief Zimunya's village in 1893, but died shortly afterward.[55] Therefore, the first real medical mission services to be given by a doctor began in 1893 when Dr. W. L. Thompson, an American Board missionary, opened a dispensary at his house in Mt. Selinda in southeastern Zimbabwe. Dr. Thompson was later joined by Dr. W. T. Lawrence in 1900, who founded a small hospital at Chikore, 15 miles west of Mt. Selinda. Another early practitioner was Samuel Gurney of the American Methodist Episcopal Church who started providing medical services to Africans at Old Mutare in March 1903.[56]

The American Board Mission played a vital role in the health delivery systems of both Zimbabwe and Mozambique. Its main station at Mt. Selinda was established in 1893. Although the missionary physician, Dr. Thompson, reported in 1894 that the medical work of the mission station was still small, with about two cases daily, including white patients, he was confident that this work would increase with time.[57]

The medical missionaries dealt with a wide range of diseases and conditions among both Africans and white settlers. The most common disease was malaria. Other diseases included syphilis, intestinal worms, skin infections, eye and ear infections, diarrhea, dysentery, enteritis, respiratory infections, and gynecological infections. The missionaries reported that they had attended to approximately 590 cases in 1894.[58] Of these cases, 268 were African while 94 were among white settlers.

With little government medical infrastructure available, colonial governments depended on the American Board Mission to provide health services to Africans as well as to white settlers in this southern portion of the Zimbabwe-Mozambique border region where the American Board Mission station was located. This was shown by the willingness of colonial

[55] Gelfand, *A Service to the Sick*, 100.

[56] Ibid.

[57] ABC 15.4 volume 19: Letter from W. L. Thompson, Mt. Selinda to Judson Smith, Boston, MA, April 6, 1894.

[58] ABC 15.4 volume 20: Letter from W. L. Thompson, Mt. Selinda to E. E. Strong, Boston, MA, February 18, 1895.

governments, particularly that of Zimbabwe, to fund medical missionaries. In view of the fact that they were providing medical services to European settlers, the American Board requested medical aid from the colonial government in Zimbabwe as early as 1896.[59] In 1908, the missionaries received a horse from the government for the use of their Medical Department.[60] The horse helped missionary physicians visit white patients who could not be brought to the mission for treatment. Thus, the concern of the colonial government during this early period remained exclusively on providing health care for Europeans.

During these early years, much of the assistance missionaries received from the Colonial Zimbabwean Government for the provision of African health care was in the form of free medicines. In 1911 the government supplied free remedies for the treatment of syphilis and had thus assisted the missionaries in coping with what they thought was a "grave malady ... so prevalent among the natives."[61] However, two years later, the Medical Director recommended that six missionary physicians be appointed and paid by the government to take care of the health of Africans and the American Board Mission applied for one of these appointments, which the government approved.[62] Although these efforts to extend medical services to Africans were significant, they still were largely inadequate for the region.

Reflecting their principal goal of making converts, the missionaries were willing to provide medical services to the entire region and often traveled long distances to visit patients in both Zimbabwe and Mozambique. After

[59] ABC 15.4, volume 20: Letter from H.J. Gilson, Secretary, East Central Africa Mission, to Judson Smith, Secretary, ABCFM., Boston, MA., September 24th, 1896. The "unsettled state of affairs" probably involved Zimbabwe's rebellion against colonial rule, often referred to as the "First Chimurenga."

[60] ABC 15.4, volume 23: Report of the Medical Department, Rhodesian Branch, A.B.M. in S.A., June 31, 1907 to June 31, 1908. The granting of the horse was a result of a request made by white farmers and the missionaries so that Dr. Thompson could "more easily meet the [medical] needs of the district." However, the horse died in April 1913 due to horse sickness, making long trip to patients difficult to accomplish.

[61] ABC 15.4, volume 32: Annual Report, Rhodesian Branch American Board Mission in South Africa for the year ended May 31, 1911. It was a Rhodesian policy to offer treatment for venereal diseases such as syphilis free of charge to Africans. The missionaries reported later in the 1914 annual report that the government had continued to supply medicine for syphilis but the promise of 22 pounds of quinine for routine prophylactic administration "to our school children [had] not been kept, though the Medical Director expressed much interest in the experiment as already tried on a small scale."

[62] ABC 15.4, volume 32: Annual Report, Rhodesian Branch American Board Mission in South Africa for the year ended May 31, 1913.

the death of the Chipinge district surgeon in 1902, Dr. W. T. Lawrence, a missionary physician, was the "only medical man in the [Chipinge] district" embarking on long journeys to attend English, Dutch, Portuguese, or African patients.[63] As Dr. Lawrence reported in 1911, the nearest government district surgeon in Zimbabwe was 65 miles north of Mt. Selinda. Contrary to Langson Mahoso's assertion that "everyone who was sick had to come to the mission station" for treatment, the medical missionaries traveled long distances to attend to cases in both Zimbabwe and Mozambique.[64] In 1911, for example, a missionary physician traveled from Mt. Selinda, Zimbabwe, to Spungabera, Mozambique, to treat an African chief who had a heart condition and advanced tuberculosis on both lungs.[65] The cross-border nature of the American Board Mission was also shown in missionary responses to the 1918 influenza epidemic. When Spanish influenza hit these two colonies, the missionaries engaged in cross-border work of inoculating Africans.[66]

While missionary medical services for Africans were limited by the availability of resources up to the 1920s, the government finally became aware of the need to extend health services to rural Africans. This coincided with many requests for more church involvement in African health. In 1924 Reverend Dr. Samuel Gurney of the United Methodist Church advocated the unity of the two phases of mission work, preaching and medicine, claiming that Jesus Christ was "a medical missionary."[67] Then in 1927, the government encouraged missionary societies to engage more extensively in medical work by the payment of definite and fixed government grants toward the salaries of qualified medical missionaries and nurses and toward the maintenance of mission hospitals and dispensaries.[68]

In colonial Zimbabwe, therefore, Government Notice No. 335 of 1927 introduced "one of the Administration's most significant and progressive health measures" by legalizing the payment of grants to missionary societies that provided medical attention to Africans in the tribal trust lands

[63] ABC 15.4, volume 25: Letter from H. J. Gilson, Melsetter, Rhodesia to The Prudential Committee of the ABCFM, Boston, MA, December 29th, 1902.

[64] Langson Takawira Mahoso, "The Social Impact of Christian Missions in Zimbabwe 1900–1930: A case Study of American Board Mission, Brethren in Christ Mission and the Seventh Day Adventist Mission," M.A. Thesis (Temple University, 1979), 31.

[65] ABC 15.4, volume 32: Report Letter No. 20 from the Mt. Silinda Station, American Board Mission in South Africa, Rhodesian Branch, April 12, 1911.

[66] See Dube, "Medicine without Borders."

[67] NAZ, S1173/301–304, "Health and the Native," Rhodesia Herald, June 5, 1924.

[68] NAZ, S1173/328–329, Medical Director to Colonial Secretary, June 9, 1927.

(reserves).[69] The grants would be used to pay the salaries of medical missionaries and nurses, for the maintenance of African hospitals, for the establishment of training schools for African probationer nurses (later known as nursing assistants) of either sex, and for the purchase of drugs and dressings for the upkeep of outdoor dispensaries.

On the Mozambican side of the border, there was negligible government aid. Yet the missionaries still engaged in cross-border work, treating Africans in local contexts. Thus the ever-parsimonious Mozambique Company invested little in the limited medical facilities for Africans to the extent that even in the late 1920s, the hospital in Manica was described as a "'frigid cement space,' more a holding pen than an infirmary."[70] Neither did the Mozambique Company do much to assist medical missions. According to the American Board missionaries, the only help they received from the Portuguese government was the lymph used to administer about 150 vaccinations for smallpox between 1933 and 1934.[71] As for the rest of Mozambique, Allen and Barbara Isaacman put it succinctly when they wrote that in Mozambique the Portuguese set up medicine and education to serve the privileged white settler community, with an absolute lack of health care facilities in the rural areas, where the majority of the African population lived.[72]

Consequently, there was even greater dependence on missionary medicine in Mozambique in the provision of health services for rural Africans. The Mossurize district administrator reported in 1933 that some Africans utilized the American Board Mission Hospital at Mount Selinda, "where they have a good American doctor and two or three nurses of the same nationality."[73] He also asserted that at the American Board satellite dispensary at the Bela Vista School in Gogoyo, an American nurse gave good

[69] Gelfand, *A Service to the Sick*, 116.

[70] Allina, *Slavery By Any Other Name*, 57.

[71] ABC 15.6, volume 2: Reports, 1930–1939—Gogoi Medical Report, June 1933–June 1934. Dr. W. T. Lawrence resigned from the American Board Mission in May 1946. Mission secretary D. U. Marsh wrote to the Registrar of the Medical Council of Southern Rhodesia in March 1946 informing him of the retirement of Dr. Lawrence. The Mission was unable to secure a doctor to replace him and this left its "native medical work of 50 years standing in a difficult position." See NAZ, S2014/6/3: The American Board Mission, 1925–1947—Letter from D. U. Marsh, Secretary of the American Board Mission, Mount Selinda, to the Registrar of the Medical Council of Southern Rhodesia, March 30th, 1946.

[72] Isaacman and Isaacman, *Mozambique*, 52–53.

[73] AHM, FCM, Secretaria Geral—Relatórios: Report of the District of Mossurize—Health Services, 1933, box no. 265, file no. 5821. My translations.

medical services.[74] In addition, in 1935, the administrator reported that medical assistance to indigenous people was provided by local Post Administrators who used ambulances to transport some African patients to the Mt. Selinda hospital.[75] The American nurse probably encouraged patients to consult mission doctors at Mt. Selinda, whereas the administrator of the district disliked movement across the border. The missionaries at Mt. Selinda claimed that patients came from all directions and often traveled 50 or even 100 miles in order to reach the hospital. A particular case was that of a young man who came from a village in Mozambique, 50 miles away from Mt. Selinda, suffering from a broken back and complete paralysis, the result of an accident in a mine shaft in Johannesburg, South Africa.[76]

In Mozambique, therefore, just as in Zimbabwe, rural health services were left to missionaries and these services were inadequate. The ideal solution, according to the administrator, was constructing a small ward for the indigenous people of Upper Mossurize in order to reduce their dependence on Mt. Selinda.[77] The Mozambique Company finally established a clinic at Spungabera around 1940, two years before the Company ceased governing Mozambique.

By the 1950s, there was only one hospital at Macequece, serving the districts of Manica, Mossurize, and Moribane.[78] It catered mostly for the European population and Africans employed in public works. To the south, in the Mossurize district (with an estimated population of 38,183

[74] Ibid.

[75] AHM, FCM, Secretaria Geral—Relatórios: Report of the District of Mossurize for the Year 1935. Box no. 266.

[76] ABC 15.6, volume 9: Institutions—Mt. Selinda Hospital, Annual Report, 1944. It was common for young men from Mozambique to go to work in the South African mines, but this also shows the neglect that migrant miners faced from mining companies in South Africa. These mining companies simply sent the sick and injured back to their villages and recruit new healthy workers. This was particularly the case with those workers who contracted tuberculosis on the mines. See Packard, *White plague, Black Labor* and Susan Parnell, "Creating Racial Privilege: The Origins of South African Public Health and Town Planning Legislation," *Journal of Southern African Studies*, 19 (1993) 471–488.

[77] AHM, FCM, Secretaria Geral—Relatórios: Report of the District of Mossurize for the Year 1935. Box no. 266.

[78] AHM, FCM, Secretaria Geral—Relatórios, Macequece, August, 1904, Caixa 126, Pasta 26636.

Africans in 1938),[79] there was only one clinic at Spungabera and another at Chibabava. Some of the medical facilities were in the Mozambique Company's schools, serving as posts to distribute medicines. However, there were barely any health services provided for Africans in the Moribane district, falling between Mossurize to the south and Manica to the north. The Portuguese neglected this district to the extent that it became a backward post and an undeclared labor reserve.[80]

In colonial Zimbabwe, however, as the government sought to rely more on missionaries for the provision of medical services to Africans in rural areas, some health officials were concerned about how, in their view, missionaries easily accommodated African preference for out-patient treatment instead of confining Africans in hospitals. In colonial Zimbabwe, for instance, the Medical Director raised concerns about the provision of medicines to Africans, at government expense, by missionaries, who argued that Africans disliked hospitals and the out-patient system of health care was the most effective way treating them.[81] He therefore recommended that missionary societies accepting government grants should consent to government inspection and the right to call for any reports and returns in order to "keep a modicum of control in the hands of the Government."

Without any input into the treatment process, many African villagers thought that treatment in government hospitals was another form of submission to colonial authority. One village elder, Mr. T. Mbekwa, recalled that most Africans, particularly the elders, did not visit hospitals when sick because they thought that avoiding the hospital was a way of resisting the colonial governments and their westernizing influence.[82]

However, merely distributing medicines to African villagers was sometimes not enough to convert them. Villagers were not easily swayed by Western medicine because they had great confidence in their own medicine. The missionaries complained, "so great is the confidence they [Africans] feel in the native witch doctor, that they are liable to go to him rather than to the physician, or else to use the treatment of both at the

[79] AHM, FCM, Secretaria Geral—Relatórios: Relatório da circunscrição de Mossurize referente ao Ano de 1938, Caixa 266.

[80] Allina, *Slavery By Any Other Name*, 140.

[81] NAZ, S1173/328–329, Medical Director to Colonial Secretary, June 9, 1927.

[82] Interview with Mr. T. Mbekwa, Mpanyeya, Mozambique, 14 December, 2006. Although this interviewee links African resistance to hospitalization with colonialism, most elderly people probably thought they would just die in hospitals.

same time."[83] One of the physicians noted that the Africans wanted "quick results" and that they sometimes got them from African healers.[84] African villagers thought Western medicine was inferior because those treated in hospitals took much time to recover. For Africans who wanted quick results, Western medicines proved ineffective and unnecessary.[85]

In addition, some Africans believed that they would not recover in hospitals. Dr. Lawrence noted that Africans were very afraid of being treated in a hospital. "Boys at work in the mines and towns," he claimed, "frequently run away when ill or maimed rather than subject themselves to hospital treatment. They say that if a sick native does not get well soon, the attendants give him poison to put him to sleep and he never awakens!"[86] Many interviewees confirmed the complaints of missionary physicians that Africans thought they would be "finished off" or killed if they sought treatment in hospitals. One recalled, "My uncle died in the hospital after his daughter forced him to go there. So, after his death, the whole clan did not entertain the idea of going to hospitals because they thought that hospital personnel killed patients they did not like."[87] Another recalled that there were rumors that the white people had brought drugs to inject and kill children. Thus, when Portuguese authorities announced they would "inject children in schools to prevent some diseases, many parents stopped sending their children to school."[88]

Rumors of killings in hospitals resulted from mortality in hospitals and perceived ineffectiveness of Western medicine. In most cases Africans tried traditional healers first before consulting Western doctors. They then took the patient to the hospital as a last resort when he or she was critically ill. When that patient died in the hospital, Africans then thought the hospital personnel had "finished off" that patient. One interviewee said that "even today, those who have knowledge of traditional medicines would try to help themselves first, before going to the hospital."[89]

[83] ABC 15.4, volume 32: "General Letter in regard to the Work of the Rhodesia Branch of the American Board Mission in South Africa," May 1910.

[84] Ibid.

[85] Interview, Maengeni Village, Zimbabwe, 14 January, 2007.

[86] ABC 15.4 volume 33: Letter from Dr. W. T. Lawrence, Mt. Selinda, to Rev. J. E. Burton, Secretary ABCFM, Boston, MA, October 6th, 1916.

[87] Interview, Beacon Hill, Chipinge District, Zimbabwe, 29 December, 2006.

[88] Interview, Zangiro, Mozambique, 23 September, 2006.

[89] Interview, Zimunya District, Mutare South, Zimbabwe, 31 July, 2006.

Similar views on death in colonial hospitals could be found in other parts of Africa. During the first four decades of colonial rule in Kenya, for example, where the Public Health Act required hospitals to dispose a corpse if the immediate relatives did not claim the body, there were fears about death and disappearance of bodies in hospitals. This was a period when hospitals were relatively few and did not have basic facilities such as mortuaries, with high death rates that at times were over 100 per 1000 admissions.[90] However, as George Ndege pondered, how could it be explained to people that "specimens were collected too late, that the diagnosis was completed too late or was inaccurate, and that when a patient died in a makeshift hospital the state was forced to dispose of the body because the relatives did not arrive in time to claim it for a culturally correct burial ceremony"?[91] This contributed to distrust by highlighting the perils of confinement in hospitals and the dangers of laboratories.

As the Kenyan case shows, the establishment of hospitals thus gave rise to anxieties over the impression that the majority of the people who went to the hospital for treatment were brought back dead, or never seen again, as two critical factors came together: death and the disappearance of bodies.[92] Ndege adds that apart from looking suspicious, without the requisite burial rites and rituals, hasty burials contradicted cultural tradition.[93] In Zimbabwe, villagers were afraid of dying in hospitals and being buried by *mabhanditi*/"bandits" (prisoners) in government-issued metal caskets far away from home. Africans resented these "pauper burials" in which people were buried naked.[94] In Mozambique, the Director of the Mozambique Company's Native Labor Department observed, "the native has great repugnance for being treated by whites and much more so for entering the hospital, because they think that once they enter that place they'll never leave."[95] Hence, for many forced laborers in Mozambique, the hospital was at best a "respite (from forced labor), at worst, a place to die alone, far from home and family." Worse still, dying in the hospital resulted hasty burials in shallow graves, from which their corpses could be dug up by

[90] Ndege, *Health, State, and Society in Kenya*, 42.
[91] Ibid., 7.
[92] Ibid., 42.
[93] Ibid., 43–44.
[94] Ranger, *Bulawayo Burning*, 49.
[95] Allina, *Slavery By Any Other Name*, 58.

roaming hyenas whereas their relatives would properly bury them deep in the ground and watch over the grave if they had died at home.[96]

Another major source of distrust of hospitalization was the collection of bodily fluids, particularly blood. It has already been demonstrated in Chap. 5 that many African villagers in the Zimbabwe-Mozambique border region considered blood sacred and that the blending of blood through transfusions was considered a taboo. Yet the nineteenth-century laboratory revolution demanded the collection of a patient's bodily fluids in order to accurately diagnose disease, which "sometimes went against tradition."[97] In African societies, many believed that these fluids, particularly blood, could be manipulated to harm the individual through witchcraft. Blood was important because it defined many social and kinship relations and codes of conduct as well as therapeutic measures as it was considered "a unique, cardinal principle of life."[98] The collection of blood thus raised many questions, doubts, and myths, even when the purpose was explained and African fears were exacerbated by the fact that the blood collected was never seen again. Similar views on the sanctity of blood and fears of laboratories abound from other parts of Africa, reflecting the African distrust in Western healing. In colonial Zambia, game rangers were said to capture Africans to extract their blood, mine managers captured Africans in the Belgian Congo and kept them in pits, firefighters reportedly subdued Africans with injections in Kenya but with masks in Uganda, and Africans captured in Tanganyika "were hung upside down, their throats were cut, and their blood drained into huge buckets."[99] Thus echoing Foucauldian biopolitics, Patrick Malloy has argued that this microscopic examination of bodily tissues "not only provided a new and objective basis for the diagnoses of diseases, but also reduced the patient's body to a microscopic slide."[100]

Africans' distrust of the hospital also arose from their desire to play an active role in the healing process. They were drawing upon some aspects of the precolonial healing which granted patients and their families or "therapy managers" a high degree of control over healing. In precolonial

[96] Ibid.

[97] Ndege, *Health, State, and Society in Kenya*, 41–42.

[98] Ibid.

[99] White, *Speaking with Vampires*, 4–5.

[100] Patrick Malloy, "Research Material and Necromancy: Imagining the Political Economy of Biomedicine in Colonial Tanganyika," *International Journal of African Historical Studies* 47, 3 (2014): 425.

healing, therapy managers, usually selected from among the patient's relatives, neighbors, and friends, were at the core of African healing.[101] The roles of these therapy managers were determined only by their relationship with the patient and the patient's particular malady. It was also the responsibility of therapy managers to help choose among healers and pay for health care in some cases. Therapy management served two functions. The first was "authoritative diagnosis and control over treatment," which was the responsibility of one person (or limited group) with juridical authority over the patient.[102] This one person could be the father or the husband of the patient. However, adult men and independent women could make therapy decisions for themselves. The second function of therapy management involved supportive care, which was distributed widely among neighbors, old friends, passers-by, and distant relatives. All these could inform on possible diagnoses and treatments, but could only share in the final decisions if they were invited to do so by the authority bearers.[103]

The process of diagnosing and treating an illness in precolonial society sometimes required many players because it was complex. Ideas of disease causation and diagnosis often involved differentiating between misfortunes or diseases originating from "natural" or God-given causes from those stemming from human action.[104] Both the living and the dead (ancestors) were believed to cause disease or misfortune. Thus in the Kongo society of Central Africa, for instance, efforts to understand disorder were driven by a compelling worldview, which questioned whether or not the disorder was merely a matter of fact or whether it was caused by other persons, spirits, ancestors, or the society at large.[105] In this Kongo society ancestors represented an extension of the human community as a major cause of misfortune and cure in African society. In eastern Bantu cultures, including those of Mozambique and Zimbabwe, ancestors or spirits of the dead are known by the common term, *dimu* (which is probably proto-Bantu) and as *mudzimu* (singular) and *vadzimu* (plural) among the Shona of the Zimbabwe-Mozambique border region. Among the Shona are the *Ndau* or *VaNdau* in the southern portion of the border

[101] Steven Feierman and John M. Janzen, Introduction to *The Social Basis of Health and Healing in Africa* (Berkeley: University of California Press, 1992), 18.

[102] Ibid.

[103] Ibid.

[104] John M. Janzen, *Ngoma: Discourses of Healing in Central and Southern Africa* (Berkeley: University of California Press, 1992), 65.

[105] Ibid., 86.

region; they are considered the original ancestors of the Kalanga (a South Shona or Thonga group) and "the most powerful spirit group, with a direct interest in the affairs of the living."[106]

For many Africans, diagnosis of disease thus involved questions of *who* caused the disease, not only *what* caused it. The local social context was therefore central in the diagnosis and treatment of disease. While the *n'anga* (African healer) provided answers to both questions, Western medical physicians could not say who caused the disease. According to one interviewee,

> When the sick visited a *N'anga*, the *N'anga* would determine the cause of sickness, where the disease came from, and who bewitched the sick person. So, we, as Africans, trusted that very much, to know where the infection came from and what would happen next [the prognosis]. The *N'anga* would give all that information in addition to the treatments. So, people favored the *N'anga* because they got much information about the illness.[107]

Understanding the traditional African approach to health and healing also helps in analyzing the role of AICs. The concept of illness in African society was wide, encompassing ancestors, witches, and sorcerers. Illness was therefore attributed to an imbalance between humans and spiritual or mystical forces, and the aim of healing was to restore this balance, which was achieved through communication and communion with the ancestors by performing rites, rituals, and ceremonies.[108] However, this did not mean that African medicine was always effective. The fact that Africans were willing to try other alternatives clearly demonstrates the inadequacy of African medicine.

The spread of Christianity led to the incorporation of these religious beliefs and practices, particularly among AICs. In some of these churches, strong beliefs in the traditional healing system prevailed, with some people believed to have an inherent quality that allowed them to morph into an animal, roam invisibly, and cause death or misfortune.[109] Many Africans

[106] Ibid., 95.

[107] Interview, Mvududu Village, Mutare South, Zimbabwe, 3 August, 2006.

[108] M. V. Bührmann, "Religion and Healing: The African Experience," in *Afro-Christian Religion and Healing in Southern Africa*, ed. G. C. Oosthuizen et al., (Lewiston: The Edwin Mellen Press, 1989), 26–34.

[109] W. D. Hammond-Tooke, "The Aetiology of Spirit in Southern Africa," in *Afro-Christian Religion and Healing in Southern Africa*, ed. G. C. Oosthuizen et al., (Lewiston: The Edwin Mellen Press, 1989), 44–65.

believed that witches and sorcerers possessed malevolent powers over others that caused evil. This evil could be classified as evil incarnate (the witch) or evil inherent in matter (sorcery) and was explicitly connected to antisocial behaviors and actions that threatened the fabric of society with negative feelings of envy, jealousy, and anger.[110]

Some AICs partially adopted these traditional beliefs. For the Zionists, in particular, the real adversary was the sorcerer.[111] In these AICs, the office of prophet/prayer healer became a substitute for the office of the diviner in the African society, where most of the prophets were assisted by ancestral spirits in the diagnosis and treatment of illness.[112] For some AICs in the Zimbabwe-Mozambique border region, evil spirits and witchcraft were recognized as legitimate explanations of illness or misfortune. Like the *n'anga*, prophets in these churches could, according to some interviewees, point to who caused an illness or anomaly in a patient. One woman who could not conceive noted,

> I have once been to the Mapostori [Apostles]. I could not conceive and they helped me much. I had been to hospitals also but it did not work for me. … Maybe they [Western doctors] should even allow us to catch witches because I was told the person who was blocking my tubes and I believe it is her. I was shown so many things I did not know about healing by these African prophets, only that they mix Christianity with traditional African ways which can be confusing.[113]

The same is true for other parts of Southern Africa, for example, in South Africa, where Zulu Zionists fight the use of the *inyanga*'s (African healer's) medicines and struggle against the diviner's "demons of possession" using an arsenal of old Zulu religion.[114]

However, other AICs discouraged or disassociated themselves from the use of traditional medicine and veneration of ancestors. For instance, when South African faith healers (prophets) were asked to compare

[110] Ibid., 53.

[111] G. C. Oosthuizen, "Indigenous healing within the context of the African Independent Churches," in *Afro-Christian Religion and Healing in Southern Africa*, ed. G. C. Oosthuizen et al., (Lewiston: The Edwin Mellen Press, 1989), 71–90.

[112] Ibid.

[113] Interview, Old West Mine Compound, Penhalonga, Zimbabwe, 28 August 2006.

[114] Bengt Sundkler, *Bantu Prophets in South Africa* (Oxford: Oxford University Press, 1961), 55.

themselves with the traditional healers (diviners), they said the major distinction between prophets and diviners was that prophets attend churches, pray, and use only holy water, while diviners use herbs, bones, and "killing medicine."[115]

In contrast to the willingness of AICs to work with concepts of disease and healing, the reluctance of Western medical practitioners to learn about and understand African ideas of causation and healing partly explains non-compliance with public health. According to one interviewee, the greatest weakness of Western medicine was that it could not diagnose an illness caused by witchcraft because Western doctors did not understand it, "because of their mentality, they could not accept it."[116] Accordingly, the clinics could not diagnose and treat diseases believed to be caused by one's enemies, the witches. The same interviewee warned, "You see these diseases have their own origins and we need to be careful when we seek treatment from Western doctors because we can waste lots of money on what the *n'anga* can easily see." Another interviewee argued, "Sometimes you want to hear many views especially those that are easy to understand not those long confusing words of doctors which are hard to understand. I do not like them."[117]

When asked if Africans still go the traditional healers, one interviewee responded, "Yes, [because] some diseases caused by evil spirits and sorcery cannot be treated in hospitals."[118] That explains why some Africans consulted traditional healers first, before going to the hospital. According to one interviewee, "when Africans got sick, they always wondered if they had spirits [*mambepo*]. So, they would say, let me go to the *n'anga* first, to get rid of the spirits before going to the hospital."[119] Even African nurses encouraged African patients to consult traditional healers to determine if there was no sorcery or evil spirits involved in their illness. These nurses claimed that the patients could be treated easily at the hospital only after these evil spirits had been removed.[120] Studies in some Central African societies have also revealed that although the signs and symptoms

[115] W. H. Wessels, "Healing practices in the African Independent Churches," in *Afro-Christian Religion and Healing in Southern Africa*, ed. G. C. Oosthuizen et al. (Lewiston: The Edwin Mellen Press, 1989), 91–108.

[116] Interview, Tsvingwe Village, Penhalonga, Zimbabwe, 28 August, 2006.

[117] Interview, Elim Mission, Penhalonga, Zimbabwe, 29 August, 2006.

[118] Interview, Zimunya District, Mutare South, Zimbabwe, 31 July, 2006.

[119] Interview, Nehwangura Village, Mutare South, Zimbabwe, 2 August, 2006.

[120] Interview, Ngaone, Chipinge, Zimbabwe, 20 October, 2006.

accompanying the sick could be identified and treated using Western biomedical methods and medicine, "the salient point that brings these sufferers to diagnostic entry into the ritual therapies is not so much the sickness but the identification of the spirit force behind the sickness."[121]

Prophylactic measures against sorcery and witchcraft involved methods which Western medical practitioners dismissed as mere superstition. According to one interviewee, government and medical missionaries did not tolerate the African practice of "immunizing babies by tying *madumwa* and *mazango* [charms used to protect children from sorcery and disease]. They did not see that as useful. Treatment for them probably meant an injection [shot] not a necklace [charm] tied around the waist of a baby."[122]

Due to the complexity of ideas of causation and healing in precolonial society, the nature of illness determined approaches to diagnosis and healing. In the case of illnesses understood to be caused by malevolent powers of others (which Western practitioners did not acknowledge), it was important that healing be done in local social contexts, where patients had access to multiple therapeutic alternatives and advice from kin and where practitioners could get detailed knowledge of the particular society. This was because, unlike the ancestors, who many Africans believed could follow a person everywhere, the effective range of witchcraft was limited to a small area.[123] These illnesses sometimes entailed the intervention of traveling specialists called in from afar, just as the medical missionaries did outcalls. Thus, among some AICs, such as the Zionists of South Africa, apart from restoring physical and mental well-being, a further dimension of healing was realized when the whole Zionist congregation visited the homestead of the patient. Here, the healer played a central role in rendering the homestead safe for habitation either by removing the cause of illness or by strengthening the other occupants of the homestead and the homestead itself against any further mystical attacks.[124] This explains why some African patients who were taken out of their local social context to confinement in a distant hospital would not expect to get better.

[121] John M. Janzen, *Ngoma*, 92–93.

[122] Interview, Elim Mission, Penhalonga, Zimbabwe, 29 August, 2006.

[123] W. D. Hammond-Tooke, "The Aetiology of Spirit in Southern Africa," 53–54.

[124] D. Dube, "A Search for Abundant Life: Health, Healing and Wholeness in the Zionist Churches," in *Afro-Christian Religion and Healing in Southern Africa*, ed. G. C. Oosthuizen et al., (Lewiston: The Edwin Mellen Press, 1989), 109–136.

However, in other cases, particularly those believed to involve spirit possession, physical ailments, and misfortune, patients themselves traveled to specialists. Many spirit-type or independent churches replicated this pattern even though it often required clandestine trans-frontier movements which colonial governments sought to suppress. Colonial health practitioners and Christian missionaries in the border region commented on this pattern of health delivery, which sometimes rivaled theirs. In 1934 Gertrude Merrill, an American Board Mission nurse at Gogoyo, reported, "Mention should be made of a rival in the healing art who appeared a few months ago, who claimed to be the agent of Mary Mother of God [Maria] in distributing her benefits by means of a medicine called 'muchapi.'"[125] Merrill claimed that people came from long distances with tins and containers, which this "doctor" (Maria) put in a secret place, where she would fill them with the precious fluid ("muchapi") while all were asleep during the night. She added that this fluid was supposed to "preserve" a person's purchases and family from harm or even death. "Several imbibers of 'muchapi' were treated at Gogoi for upset stomach," she asserted, adding that the "[Portuguese] Government treated with disfavor this enterprise, and I no longer hear much about it; tho[ugh] doubtless it is still carried on, being financially much more profitable to the agent than mine to the Mission."[126] Ian Phimister has attributed the emergence of these prophetic and faith healing movements to the hardships of the 1930s, engendered by the colonial states, as discussed in Chap. 3.[127]

Although the origins of *Muchapi* or *Mucapi* remain elusive, this was an anti-witchcraft movement which swept through Malawi, Zambia, and other neighboring territories during the 1930s.[128] The essence of the *Muchapi* Movement was to coordinate the surrender of medicines and medical objects during large communal rituals, where witches would confess, and all would drink the *Muchapi* medicine communally, which was

[125] ABC 15.4, volume 43; Gogoi Medical Report, June, 1933–June, 1934.

[126] Ibid.

[127] Phimister, *An Economic and Social History of Zimbabwe*, 196–197.

[128] Audrey I. Richards, "A Modern Movement of Witch-Finders," *Africa: Journal of the International African Institute* 8, no. 4 (1935): 448. For an extensive discussion of *Mucapi*, see Max Marwick, *Sorcery in its social setting: a study of the Northern Rhodesia Ceŵa* (Manchester: Manchester University Press, 1965) and W. M. J. van Binsbergen, *Religious Change in Zambia: exploratory studies* (London: Kegan Paul International, 1981).

believed to protect the imbibers from witchcraft.[129] Hence the practitioners of *Muchapi* have been referred to as "cleansers."[130]

On the Zimbabwean side of the border region, the NC Mutare reported that the "self-styled faith healer," Mai or Mayi (Mother) Chaza, established herself in the Zimunya Native Reserve in 1956.[131] He claimed that in a matter of weeks a pole and dagga town of nearly 1000 houses mushroomed. This town later became "Guta RaJehovha," Shona for "City of God." Before starting her own church, Mai Chaza, a mother of six, was a member of the Wesleyan Methodist Church. Her followers believed that she had become ill with a chronic infection, was divorced, and "died" (went into a coma), but later "resurrected." After her "resurrection," she claimed that she met Jesus Christ and became a healer and preacher, drawing upon traditional religion and history. In other accounts, however, after Mai Chaza was revived, she became a *n'anga*, earning her living by divination and spiritual healing.[132] She founded her church in 1955 and she died in 1960. This church was particularly popular with women because it highlighted motherhood and fertility.[133]

In the same vein, the NC Mutare wondered how Mai Chaza was attracting patients of all backgrounds, including Europeans and Indians in addition to Africans, when he reported,

> It is difficult to understand how this woman, surrounded as she is by small time racketeers, and relying for the most part on tricks which are reminiscent

[129] Karen E. Fields, "Christian missionaries as anticolonial militants," *Theory and Society* 11, no. 1 (1982): 104. See also, Karen E. Fields, *Revival and Rebellion in Colonial Central Africa* (Princeton: Princeton University Press, 1985).

[130] Timothy Scarnecchia, "Mai Chaza's Guta re Jehova (City of God): healing, reproduction, and urban identity in an African Independent Church" *Journal of Southern African Studies* 23, no. 1 (1997): 97.

[131] NAZ S2827/2/2/4: Annual Report of the Native Commissioner, Umtali, for the year ended 31st December, 1956.

[132] Barbara Moss, "Holding Body and Soul Together: Women, Autonomy and Christianity in Colonial Zimbabwe," (PhD Thesis, Indiana University, 1991), 165.

[133] Kathleen E. Sheldon, *Historical Dictionary of women in Sub-Saharan Africa* (Lanham: Scarecrow Press, 2005), 137. See also, Mary-Louise Martin, "The Mai Chaza Church in Rhodesia," in *African Initiatives in Religion*, ed. David B. Barret (Nairobi, East African Publishing House, 1971), 109–121; Allan Anderson, *African reformation: African initiated Christianity in the 20th century* (Trenton: Africa World Press, 2001), 119; Rosalind I. J. Hackett, "Women and New Religious Movements in Africa," in *Religion and Gender*, ed. Ursula King (Oxford: Blackwell Publishers, 1995), 257–290; and Scarnecchia, "Mai Chaza's Guta re Jehova (City of God)".

> of pseudo-spiritualists of the past—spirit voices singing on the hilltop, ceremonies in a darkened room—retains the confidence of the hundreds who still flock to her. No specific examples of "miracle cures" are known. Women who have been declared pregnant by Mayi Chaza are still pregnant 18 months later! The child will be born when Mayi Chaza wills it! It is reported that her cure for barrenness is not very original. Women who take the cure are installed in the village and admonished not to resist "spirits" which may visit them during the night. Locally these "spirits" are dubbed "the bulls of Mayi"! An interesting fact is that she is known to [a] number [of] Europeans and Indians among her patients. A European woman suffering from cancer is said to have deserted her regular doctor and now receives treatment at the Guta r[a] Jehovah.[134]

While officials attempted to discredit Mai Chaza's healing ability, they were also dismayed by the fact that Europeans and Indians were also visiting her for treatment, perhaps demonstrating dissatisfaction and ineffectiveness of Western biomedicine. However, the main concerns among officials were political. Although the same NC reported in 1958 that Mai Chaza's sect, which had continued to function in the Zimunya Reserve and "on occasions … attracted large crowds of visitors seeking relief from physical ills," was "non-political" and caused "no harm," the government still wanted to suppress it.[135] Officials wanted to suppress the sect because it attracted "non-indigenous patients," probably Mozambicans from across the eastern border. Thus in 1959 the NC Mutare reported,

> The "Guta ra Jehova" is quite clean and orderly, though measures had to be adopted to enforce the prohibition against non-indigenous patients contained in the agreement permitting this healing centre. … All sorts of accusations have been levelled with a view to having the centre closed, but the latest, that Native foreigners continue to visit the "Guta" secretly appears on investigation to be completely false and neither Chief Zimunya nor his Council are prepared to recommend Mai Chaza's removal.[136]

[134] NAZ S2827/2/2/4: Annual Report of the Native Commissioner, Umtali, for the year ended 31st December, 1956.

[135] NAZ S2827/2/2/6: Annual Report of the Native Commissioner, Umtali, for the year ended 31st December, 1958.

[136] NAZ S2827/2/2/7: Annual Report of the Native Commissioner, Umtali, for the year ended 31st December, 1959.

As a result, the church continued to flourish. A church with this name or simply G. R. J. still operates in the Zimbabwe-Mozambique border region to this day.

However, in stark contrast to these multifaceted ways of delivering treatment in African society, colonial governments insisted on confining Africans in hospitals, as the Medical Director in colonial Zimbabwe said,

> The benefits of medical treatment in acute and dangerous illness are based on constant and not periodic medication, and though it may sound humanitarian and progressive policy to establish these local dispensaries and occasional visits from a doctor, the actual results from a medical point of view are not likely to be very great. The native who is to reap the benefits of this system, is still too primitive to take advantage of it: You cannot tell an ignorant native mother whose child is suffering from an acute and dangerous disease, that she is to give it a dose of the prescribed remedy every hour, for she does not know what an hour is, and cannot calculate the dose. I think it may be generally accepted that the maladies of indigenous and uneducated natives cannot satisfactorily be treated by European methods except under supervision, and preferably in hospitals.[137]

Yet, by confining African patients in hospitals, colonial officials denied Africans one of their main approaches to diagnosis and treatment, contributing to African distrust of Western biomedicine.

Unlike colonial governments, missionaries, in addition to treating Africans in their hospitals, also treated them in their local social contexts. Missionaries realized that public health management should not be confined by the border as shown by their cross-border work, which partly accounts for why missionaries were popular in the region.

As far as hospital treatment was concerned, interviews with Africans in the border region show that they preferred missionary hospitals. Many interviewees in Chipinge district said that if they ever had to visit a hospital, they preferred missionary to government hospitals because "hospitals like the Mt. Selinda Mission hospital had better conditions, particularly the way the nurses and white doctors treated Africans, as well as the provision of adequate food, clothing, and attention."[138] By contrast, according

[137] NAZ, S1173/328–329: Medical Assistance to Indigenous Natives in Reserves, Medical Director, Southern Rhodesia, to The Secretary, Department of the Colonial Secretary, Southern Rhodesia, 9th June, 1927.

[138] Interview, Days Hill, Chipinge District, Zimbabwe, December 13, 2006.

to some interviewees, the nurses and doctors in government hospitals "looked down upon Africans, particularly the poor and the old people."[139] These interviewees also asserted that personnel in government hospitals used harsh language to Africans and, in some cases, beat old people up. This is supported by the Council of the Federation of Native Welfare Societies in Zimbabwe which recommended "that more sympathetic consideration be given to African patients by the staff employed in the [government] hospitals" and advocated improvements in African hospitals to ensure greater comfort and convenience for African patients.[140] Standard medical practices were the same in both European and African wards, but African wards were poorly equipped to the extent that the whites, Indians, and Coloreds (bi-racial people) did not want to be treated in African wards and there was pervasive racism.[141] Even the mission hospital at Mt. Selinda had separate wards for whites and Africans, but many interviewees said they received "better" care in mission than in government hospitals.

Conclusion

While the analysis of the provision of health services for Africans in Southern Africa has focused on economic imperatives such as the need for a healthy African labor force, European settlers' fears of disease also played a central role. This is true of Mozambique and Zimbabwe and it can also be applied to the entire Southern African region. The extension of colonial health services to Africans was thus informed by European settler fears and economic imperatives rather than the concern to improve African health as an end in itself. Owing to the fact that European settlers viewed Africans as reservoirs of infection, they argued that the only way to safeguard their own health from the "infectious natives" was to treat disease in the Africans. The extension of health services to Africans in the 1930s can thus be seen as the last line of defense against the spread of disease to the settler community and the need for healthy African labor force. As a

[139] Interview, Maengeni Village, Chipinge District, Zimbabwe, 14 January, 2007.

[140] NAZ S2803/FNWS/61 Internal Affairs-Hospitals, 22nd March 1943–22nd June 1950, Secretary for Native Affairs, to the Medical Director, Southern Rhodesia, 22nd March 1943.

[141] For more on racism in Mozambique Company hospitals, see Kathleen Sheldon, "Creating an Archive of Working Women's Oral Histories in Beira, Mozambique," in *Contesting Archives: Finding Women in the Sources*, ed. Napur Chaudhuri, Sherry J. Katz, and Mary Elizabeth Perry (Urbana: University of Illinois Press, 2010), 201.

result, public health policy and its modes of delivery failed to respond to African preferences.

While most Africans were hostile to intrusive public health campaigns, they were willing to experiment with the curative aspects of biomedicine, particularly out-patient treatment, which gave them a high degree of control over the healing process. Africans generally disliked confinement in hospitals which took away their ability to control the treatment process. However, colonial governments' insistence on hospitalization denied Africans one of their principal approaches to diagnosis and healing. Hence, some African patients taken out of their local social contexts to be confined in a distant hospital did not expect to get better. Practitioners on the ground, such as medical missionaries, realized that public health management should extend beyond the border to reach out to Africans in their local contexts. This partially explains why they were relatively popular among Africans.

African societies were thus open to innovation but the discriminatory nature and ineffectiveness of colonial medical services discouraged the adoption of biomedicine. Discrimination against Africans by medical personnel in government hospitals contributed to African distrust. Colonial hospitals were highly segregated and Africans received second-grade care while confined in these hospitals. It is not surprising, therefore, that Africans preferred treatment from medical missionaries, who usually distributed medicines and instructions on their use, leaving the whole treatment process in African hands.

Finally, there was a general lack of effort on the part of colonial governments to learn about African understandings of disease causation and healing. The colonial paternalistic doctrine meant that Europeans mostly dismissed African knowledge systems as dangerous superstition. This was reinforced by the various borders and tiers of health care provision within these colonies.

References

Allina, Eric. *Slavery By Any Other Name: African Life Under Company Rule in Colonial Mozambique*. Charlottesville: University of Virginia Press, 2012.

Anderson, Allan. *African Reformation: African Initiated Christianity in the 20th Century*. Trenton: Africa World Press, 2001.

Baronov, David. *The African Transformation of Western Medicine and the Dynamics of Global Cultural Exchange*. Philadelphia: Temple University Press, 2008.

Bastos, Cristiana. "Medical Hybridisms and Social Boundaries: Aspects of Portuguese Colonialism in Africa and India in the Nineteenth Century." *Journal of Southern African Studies* 33, no. 4 (2007): 767–782.

Beck, Ann. *A Medical History of the British Medical Administration of East Africa, 1900–1950*. Cambridge: Harvard University Press, 1970.

Binsbergen, W. M. J. van. *Religious Change in Zambia: Exploratory Studies*. London: Kegan Paul International, 1981.

Bührmann, M. V. "Religion and Healing: The African Experience." In *Afro-Christian Religion and Healing in Southern Africa*, edited by G. C. Oosthuizen et al. 26–34. Lewiston: The Edwin Mellen Press, 1989.

Burton, Andrew and Michael Jennings. "The Emperor's New Clothes?: Continuities in Governance in Late Colonial and Early Post colonial East Africa." *International Journal of African Historical Studies* 40, no. 1 (2007): 1–25.

Dube, D. "A Search for Abundant Life: Health, Healing and Wholeness in the Zionist Churches." In *Afro-Christian Religion and Healing in Southern Africa*, edited by G. C. Oosthuizen et al. 109–136. Lewiston: The Edwin Mellen Press, 1989.

Dube, Francis. "Medicine without Borders: the American Board of Commissioners for Foreign Missions in central Mozambique and eastern Zimbabwe, 1893–1920s." *OFO: Journal of Transatlantic Studies* 4, no. 2 (2014): 21–38.

Feierman, Steven and John M. Janzen. Introduction to *The Social Basis of Health and Healing in Africa*. Berkeley: University of California Press, 1992.

Fields, Karen E. "Christian Missionaries as Anticolonial Militants." *Theory and Society* 11, no. 1 (1982): 95–108.

Fields, Karen E. *Revival and Rebellion in Colonial Central Africa*. Princeton: Princeton University Press, 1985.

Foucault, Michel. *Discipline and Punish: The Birth of the Prison*. New York: Vintage Books, 1995.

Gelfand, Michael. *Proud Record in Health Services in Rhodesia and Nyasaland*. Salisbury, Southern Rhodesia, 1959.

Hackett, Rosalind I. J. "Women and New Religious Movements in Africa." In *Religion and Gender*, edited by Ursula King. 257–290. Oxford: Blackwell Publishers, 1995.

Hammond-Tooke, W. D., "The Aetiology of Spirit in Southern Africa." In *Afro-Christian Religion and Healing in Southern Africa*, edited by G. C. Oosthuizen et al. 44–65. Lewiston: The Edwin Mellen Press, 1989.

Isaacman, Allen and Isaacman, Barbara. *Mozambique: From Colonialism to Revolution, 1900–1982*. Boulder: Westview Press, 1983.

Janzen, John M.. *Ngoma: Discourses of Healing in Central and Southern Africa*. Berkeley: University of California Press, 1992.

Kaler, Amy. "The White Man in the Bedroom: Contraception and Resistance on Commercial Farms in Colonial Rhodesia." In *Biomedicine as a Contested Site: Some Revelations in Imperial Contexts*, edited by Poonam Bala. 79–98. Lanham, MD: Lexington Books, 2009.

Lachenal, Guillaume. "A Genealogy of Treatment as Prevention (TasP): Prevention, Therapy, and the Tensions of Public Health in African History." In *Global Health in Africa: Historical Perspectives on Disease*, edited by James L. A. Webb, JR. and Tamara Giles-Vernick. 70–91. Athens: Ohio University Press, 2013.

Lewis, Joanna. *Empire State-Building: War And Welfare In Kenya 1925–1952.* Athens: Ohio University Press, 2001.

Mahoso, Langson Takawira. "The Social Impact of Christian Missions in Zimbabwe 1900–1930: A case Study of American Board Mission, Brethren in Christ Mission and the Seventh Day Adventist Mission." M.A. Thesis, Temple University, 1979.

Malloy, Patrick. "Research Material and Necromancy: Imagining the Political Economy of Biomedicine in Colonial Tanganyika." *International Journal of African Historical Studies* 47, no. 3 (2014): 425–443.

Martin, Mary-Louise. "The Mai Chaza Church in Rhodesia." In *African Initiatives in Religion*, edited by David B. Barret. 109–121. Nairobi, East African Publishing House, 1971.

Marwick, Max. *Sorcery in Its Social Setting: A Study of the Northern Rhodesia Cewa.* Manchester: Manchester University Press, 1965.

Moss, Barbara. "Holding Body and Soul Together: Women, Autonomy and Christianity in Colonial Zimbabwe." PhD Thesis, Indiana University, 1991.

Ndege, George O. *Health, State, and Society in Kenya.* Rochester: University of Rochester Press, 2001.

Oosthuizen, G. C. "Indigenous Healing Within the Context of the African Independent Churches." In *Afro-Christian Religion and Healing in Southern Africa*, edited by G. C. Oosthuizen, S. D. Edwards, W. H. Wessels, and Irving Hexham. 71–90. Lewiston: The Edwin Mellen Press, 1989.

Packard, Randall M. *White Plague, Black Labor: Tuberculosis and the Political Economy of Health and Disease in South Africa.* Berkeley: University of California Press, 1989.

Packard, Randall M.. "Visions of Postwar Health and Development and Their Impact on Public Health Interventions in the Developing World." In *Internal Development and the Social Sciences: Essays on the History and Politics of Knowledge*, edited by Fredrick Cooper and Randall Packard. 93–115. Berkeley: University of California Press, 1997.

Parnell, Susan. "Creating Racial Privilege: The Origins of South African Public Health and Town Planning Legislation." *Journal of Southern African Studies*, 19 (1993): 471–488.

Phimister, Ian. *An Economic and Social History of Zimbabwe, 1890–1948: Capital Accumulation and Class Struggle*. London: Longman, 1988.
Prince, Ruth J. "Introduction: Situating Health and the Public in Africa." In *Making and Unmaking of Public Health in Africa: Ethnographic and Historical Perspectives*, edited by Ruth J. Prince and Rebecca Marsland. 1–51. Athens: Ohio University Press, 2014.
Ranger, Terence. *Bulawayo Burning: The Social History of a Southern African City, 1893–1960*. James Currey: Suffolk, 2010.
Richards, Audrey I. "A Modern Movement of Witch-Finders." *Africa: Journal of the International African Institute* 8, no. 4 (1935): 448–461.
Scarnecchia, Timothy. "Mai Chaza's Guta re Jehova (City of God): Healing, Reproduction, and Urban Identity in an African Independent Church." *Journal of Southern African Studies* 23, no. 1 (1997): 87–105.
Sheldon, Kathleen. *Historical Dictionary of Women in Sub-Saharan Africa*. Lanham: Scarecrow Press, 2005.
Sheldon, Kathleen. "Creating an Archive of Working Women's Oral Histories in Beira, Mozambique." In *Contesting Archives: Finding Women in the Sources*, edited by Napur Chaudhuri, Sherry J. Katz, and Mary Elizabeth Perry. 192–210. Urbana: University of Illinois Press, 2010.
Smith, Judson. *A History of the American Board Missions in Africa*. Boston, MA: American Board of Commissioners for Foreign Missions Congregational House, 1905.
Sundkler, Bengt. *Bantu Prophets in South Africa*. London: International African Institute, 1961.
Tilley, Helen. *Africa as a Living Laboratory: Empire, Development, and the Problem of Scientific Knowledge, 1870–1950*. Chicago: University of Chicago Press, 2011.
Viljoen, Russell Stafford. "Disease. Doctors and De Beers Capitalists: Smallpox and Scandal in Colonial Kimberley (South Africa) during the Mineral Revolutions and British Imperialism, c. 1882–1883." In *Biomedicine as a Contested Site: Some Revelations in Imperial Contexts*, edited by Poonam Bala. 153–169. Lanham, MD: Lexington Books, 2009.
Wessels, W. H. "Healing practices in the African Independent Churches." In *Afro-Christian Religion and Healing in Southern Africa*, ed. G. C. Oosthuizen et al. 91–108. Lewiston: The Edwin Mellen Press, 1989.
White, Luise. *Speaking with Vampires: Rumor and History in Colonial Africa*. Berkeley: University of California Press, 2000.
Worboys, Michael. "The Colonial World as Mission and Mandate: Leprosy and Empire, 1900–1940." *Osiris* 15, no. 1 (2000): 207–219.

CHAPTER 9

Conclusion

It is clear that the conjunction of a particular colonized society, a distinctive kind of colonialism, and a particular territorial border generated reluctance to embrace public health because certain colonial circumstances impeded the acceptance of therapeutic alternatives that were in fact embraced by colonized people elsewhere. Historians could look elsewhere for similar kinds of histories involving racialized application of public health policies in borderlands.

The Zimbabwe-Mozambique border was productive in many respects. The border produced not only the obvious obstructions and frustrations but also desires and needs to cross it. It produced opportunity as well as prohibition, disrupting all manner of networks of interdependence, including those of kinship in particular. The border tore apart families, and given that decisions about therapy alternatives before the establishment of the border were made collectively by groups of kin, the border made health management difficult. Travel before the advent of the border was a way of maintaining and/or regaining health, among other things. Villagers traveled to see healers, to obtain medicines, and to visit shrines of spirit mediums. Hence, the restrictions that the border imposed on movement were harmful to health. They led to low compliance, especially given that these cross-border movements were controlled by governments that were considered oppressive, exploitative, discriminatory, and unresponsive to the popular will.

However, African villagers were not simply rejecting Western medicine *per se*. There was a clear distinction between modes of treatment that they

F. Dube, *Public Health at the Border of Zimbabwe and Mozambique, 1890–1940*, African Histories and Modernities,
https://doi.org/10.1007/978-3-030-47535-2_9

accepted and those that they rejected, for example out-patient treatment versus hospitalization, respectively. This partially explains why the out-patient-focused missionary medicine was more enthusiastically welcomed than state medicine, which emphasized confinement and surveillance.

The border, which itself was created by colonial powers, became a major obstacle to the implementation of comprehensive regional public health programs. Although the border was drawn along the crest of the Vumba and Chimanimani mountains, it still arbitrarily divided a region which shared similar cultural and epidemiological characteristics. It also divided people of common origins. Thus cross-border movements, which even became more widespread due to colonial demands and African desires, had important implications for the epidemiologys of infectious and communicable diseases.

In the case of diseases such as trypanosomiasis, the border prevented the continuation of the forms of transhumance which had contributed to protecting cattle in precolonial times. In Mozambique, where Portuguese officials subjected Africans to forced labor, including wild rubber collection, colonial demands increased African susceptibility to and incidence of sleeping sickness. Here, the border also served to increase dependence on migrant labor to South Africa, because Africans could not freely seek employment or trading opportunities in Zimbabwe. In addition, colonial disruption of precolonial trypanosomiasis control methods and subsequent colonial land-use patterns contributed to an increase in the prevalence of the disease. Unlike, precolonial ways of managing trypanosomiasis, colonial measures imposed great restrictions, demanded the wholesale destruction of flora and fauna, and placed Africans and their cattle in tsetse-infested areas to act as buffer zones for Europeans and their cattle. Tsetse fly and trypanosomiasis control measures therefore disrupted the African way of life and caused much suffering. These public health and veterinary measures ultimately led to low compliance with Western medicine.

Similarly, European attitudes toward Africans affected the formulation and implementation of public health policies in the region. Erroneous views on the epidemiology of STDs by the settler community resulted in the adoption of discriminatory practices that affected the way Africans perceived public health. The colonial governments singled out Africans for intrusive medical examinations as a result of unfounded or highly exaggerated settler fears and economic considerations. Though ineffective, these policies caused hardship among Africans, from villagers, cattle keepers, and town dwellers to local and foreign labor migrants. Public pressure from white settlers, particularly in Zimbabwe, compelled public health officials to enforce intrusive public health policies, which contributed to low compliance with Western medicine. Settler fears of infection in Zimbabwe were amplified by the imagination of the border, which engendered fear of an unfamiliar "other territory" (Mozambique), which in reality was not far away.

While there were other factors that discouraged Africans from embracing Western medicine, invasive and discriminatory colonial public health policies were at the center of this reluctance in some circles of the African society. This was particularly so for the illiterate and less educated country folks. For many of these Africans, their first encounter with Western biomedicine was through these compulsory and intrusive public health campaigns, such as smallpox vaccinations. What made the experience worse was that colonial officials did little to teach or explain what they were doing to Africans. The colonial paternalistic mentality dictated that these colonial officials just tell Africans they had to submit to public health measures because these officials supposedly know what was good for Africans. It is not surprising, therefore, that when Africans think of colonial public health, they often link it to oppression. Thus, resistance to colonial public health policy and its modes of delivery became part of the general resistance to colonial domination.

The legitimacy of colonial governments was also central as effective public health compliance required trust in government. That reluctance to embrace public health resulted from lack of trust, and fear, of government institutions has been shown by contrasting low compliance with public health and willingness to benefit from curative biomedicine, which did not require the same level of trust in government. Thus, while public health measures were bound to incite resistance wherever they were implemented, their application in colonies was unusual because of colonial rule and the racial discrimination that accompanied them. Although some colonial officials argued that public health measures were implemented to benefit Africans, the primary motive behind public health policy was European settlers' health, not African health. If colonial officials were concerned with the health of Africans, they would have invested some time to learn about African understandings of disease and health. The ineffectiveness and impacts of colonial public health in the Zimbabwe-Mozambique borderland were also glaring because European settlers' fears of diseases and economic imperatives contributed to the institution of bogus public health measures which created low compliance with Western medicine among Africans.

Index[1]

[1] Note: Page numbers followed by 'n' refer to notes.

F. Dube, *Public Health at the Border of Zimbabwe and Mozambique, 1890–1940*, African Histories and Modernities,
https://doi.org/10.1007/978-3-030-47535-2

T

The manufacturer's authorised representative in the EU is Springer Nature Customer Service Centre GmbH, Europaplatz 3, 69115 Heidelberg, Germany. If you have any concerns regarding our products, please contact ProductSafety@springernature.com

Printed and bound by CPI Group (UK) Ltd, Croydon, CR0 4YY
05/10/2026
02228125-0008